GENETICS - RESEARCH AND ISSUES

MOLECULAR GENETICS OF CHRONIC PANCREATITIS AND IMPLICATIONS IN DIAGNOSIS AND PROGNOSIS

GENETICS - RESEARCH AND ISSUES

Additional books in this series can be found on Nova's website under the Series tab.

Additional e-books in this series can be found on Nova's website under the e-book tab.

GENETICS - RESEARCH AND ISSUES

MOLECULAR GENETICS OF CHRONIC PANCREATITIS AND IMPLICATIONS IN DIAGNOSIS AND PROGNOSIS

SHWETA SINGH
AND
BECHAN SHARMA

NOVA BIOMEDICAL

New York

Library of Congress Cataloging-in-Publication Data

ISBN: 978-1-63321-881-9

Library of Congress Control Number: 2014948901

Published by Nova Science Publishers, Inc. † New York

CONTENTS

PREFACE

Chronic pancreatitis (CP), a well-known global disease, is primarily recognized as a long-standing inflammation of the pancreas that alters the organ's normal structure and functions. CP is reflects the end-stage pathology of inflammation-associated diseases. It presents episodes of acute inflammation or chronic damage of pancreas with symptoms of persistent abdominal pain or malabsorption, weight loss, pain related to the intake of food containing a high percentage of fats and protein. The health conditions of diabetics have been found to be deteriorated due to pancreatic damage in CP. A plethora of information has emerged in recent years in the area of pancreatitis research. The frontiers of current pancreatic research reflected on to its newer definitions, classifications, tools for investigations, animal models, insight into the molecular mechanisms of the initiation of the earliest pancreatic injury, the role of cytokines and inflammation; and attributes of genetic mutations in pancreatitis (SPINK1 CFTR, CTSB, MTHFR and ACE) etc. The topological variations of patients have been found to be associated to a different trend of pathogenesis and severity of the disease, which might be associated to relatively poor nutritional uptake and impact of other environmental factors.

Keeping these facts in view, we envisaged to bring out an updated overview on this subject in general and to present the experiment based information on tropical chronic pancreatitis (TCP) in the patients from northern part of India in particular. This publication includes different aspects of TCP such as clinical profiling in blood of TCPs, identification and analysis of different genes associated to TCP, detection of mutations in these genes using armed PCR, RFLP, electrophoresis and DNA sequencing, establishing a correlation of these mutations to the severity and pathogenesis of TCP, gene-

gene interactions, genotype-phenotype correlation (microarray analysis), screening of different probands from TCP families and establishing these mutations as specific markers for early diagnosis and prognosis of the disease.

This book is divided in eight different sections. Section 1 presents the general introduction and background of TCP. Section 2 deals with the extensive survey of literature on the subject so as to present updated information about various aspects of TCP globally and in Indian subcontinent in particular. Section 3 demonstrates the main objectives of the study to be achieved. Section 4 describes experimental design, various specific protocols, tools and techniques implied in TCP research. Section 5 explains the data obtained from the study and involves details of even minute observations. Section 6 enumerates the discussion of data, associated mechanisms as well as molecular, genetic and environmental attributes to TCP. Section 7 is dedicated to the presentation of the summary and conclusion of the entire research work conducted in the study. Section 8 includes citations and references used in this work. This book contains many specific diagrams, illustrations and presentations in simple Tables and Figures which are self explanatory so as to make any reader well versed to this subject. In addition, the specific flow charts are added to simplify the presentation. The specific molecular markers highlighted as signatures of TCP in this publication may be of great use as they could be exploited for early diagnosis and effective treatment of the disease.

We hope that this publication would be of great use to graduates, postgraduates, researchers and faculty members who are studying or practicing gastrointestinal disorders in general and TCP in particular, diagnosis and prognosis of the disease. The techniques explained in this title could be of immense use to all those working in this area. We acknowledge the TCP patients whose cooperation could help generate this useful information.

We shall deeply appreciate receiving the comments and suggestions from the readers from different parts of the globe which would help us improve the first edition of this publication.

Shweta Singh
Bechan Sharma

About the Authors

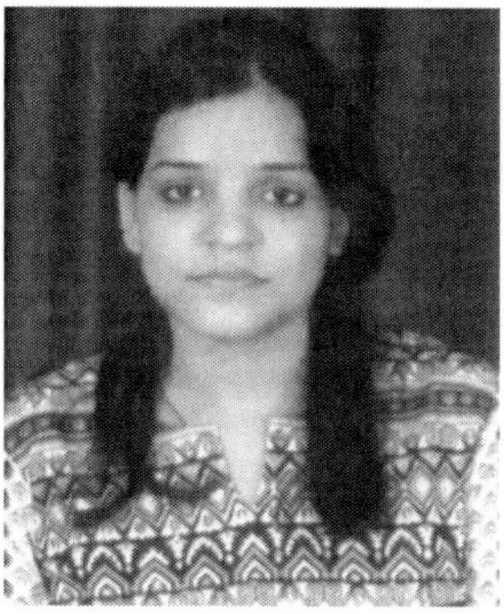

Dr. (Ms.) Shweta Singh, a gold medalist in Biochemistry from University of Allahabad, got awarded with coveted DST (ISPIRE) research fellowship. She completed her Ph.D. in Genetics from Sanjay Gandhi Post Graduate Institute of Medical Sciences-Lucknow. During her doctoral research, she received a prestigious JSPS-HOPE Fellow award at Japan. She was invited there to participate in a one week scientific congregation of Nobel Laureates. She has visited Pasteur Institute of Paris, France to participate in a ParaFrap Postdoctoral Research programme. Her area of research interest has been molecular genetics of gastrointestinal diseases in general and that of tropical chronic pancreatitis in particular. Her research interest also relates to Toxicology and oxidative stress biology. Currently, as a researcher, she is associated to the University of Rochester-NY, USA. She is the member of various national scientific bodies. She has published nine research papers in different international peer reviewed journals of repute. Her one book chapter is in print to be released by Humana Publishers, USA. She is on the panel of Reviewers for five peer reviewed international journals. She has recently been awarded with a prestigious Dr. D. S. Kothari Post Doctoral Research Fellowship by University Grants Commission, New Delhi, India to carry out research on exploring phytochemicals as antiHIV-1 therapeutics.

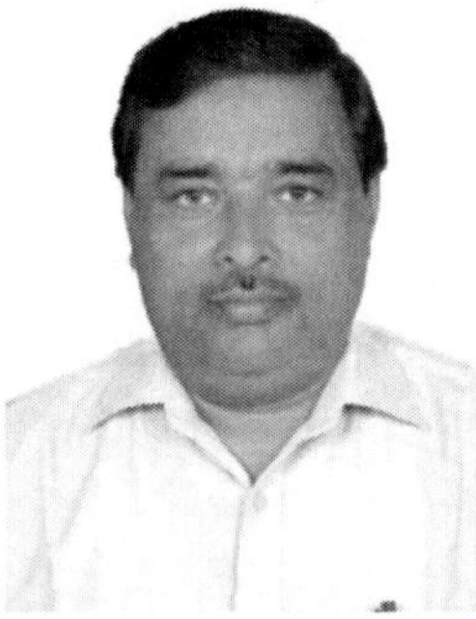

Bechan Sharma, is presently working as a Professor/Ex-Chairman, Department of Biochemistry, Allahabad University, India. He completed all his higher education from Banaras Hindu University-Varanasi, India. He carried out his doctoral research at Central Drug Research Institute-Lucknow, India. Prior to joining at University of Allahabad, he worked at Sher-Kashmir University of Agriculture Sciences and Technology–Srinagar, Kashmir (J&K) as an Assistant Professor (Veterinary Biochemistry) and Dr. RML Avadh University, Faizabad-UP as a Reader (Biochemistry). The areas of his research interests include Molecular Biology, Tropical Diseases, Phytochemistry and Toxicology. With 26 years of teaching/research experience in Biochemistry/ Biotechnology/Environmental Sciences, he has served in different capacities for many academic and administrative bodies of many Universities and Institutions. He has received number of Awards/Honors and Medals. He has produced 10 Ph.Ds. and mentored for 4 post doctoral research fellows. He has published 130 research papers, 3 Books, 12 book chapters, 3 Editorials, 3 molecular methods and several popular scientific articles in many peer reviewed international and national Journals of repute. He has one US patent. He is a member/life member of several national/international scientific societies and Fellow of Academy of Environmental Biology (FAEB)-India. He is a Lead Guest Editor of CMB-France, Natural Science (Biological Control), Natural Science (Research on Enzyme); Chief Editor of International Research Journal of Pharmacy and Pharmacology (AJPR, Academic Journals), Journal of Biochemistry Research (JBR), Sky Journal of Biochemistry Research (SJBR) and Advances in Enzyme Research (AER). He is also working as a

Guest Editor/Associate & Executive Editor/Editor-Member for 76 international Journals and as a honorary reviewer for over 120 scientific international journals of repute. He has worked as a visiting scientist in USA for 3 years and also at Italy, France, Thailand, Germany, Iran, Kuwait, Turkey and Brazil for 2-4 months where he has completed various research projects on different aspects of molecular biology of HIV-1, drug resistance in HIV-1 and *in silico* drug design and development, gene silencing and toxicology.

ABBREVIATIONS

CP	Chronic Pancreatitis
TCP	Tropical Chronic Pancreatitis
IP	Idiopathic Pancreatitis
bp	Base pair
SPINK1	Serine Protease Inhibitor Kazal Type
CFTR	Cystic Fibrosis Transmembrane Conductance Regulator
ACE	Angiotensin Converting Enzyme
PD	Pancreas Divisum
dl	Deciliter
DNA	Deoxy Ribonucleic Acid
DNTP	Dinucleotide tri phosphate
EDTA	Ethylenediamine Tetra Acetic Acid
HDL	High density lipoprotein
Hr	Hour
Kb	Kilopase pair
LDL	Low density lipoprotein
LPL	Lipoprotein lipase
M	Molar
MI	Myocardial infarction
mM	Millimolar
MTHFR	Methylenetetrahydrofolate Reductase
CTSB	Cathepsin B
OD	Optical Density
PCR	Polymerase Chain Reaction
PK	Proteinase K
pmol	Picomole

PCR	Polymerase Chain Reaction
ARMS	Amplification Refractory Mutation System
RFLP	Restriction Fragment Length Polymorphism
rpm	Revolutions per Minute
RT	Room Temperature
SDS	Sodium Dodecyl Sulphate
STE	Sodium chloride Tris EDTA
Sec	Seconds
Taq	Thermus Aquaticus DNA polymerase
TBE	Trisborate Ethylene Diamine Tetraacetic Acid
TC	Total cholesterol
TG	Triglyceride
UV	Ultraviolet
VLDL	Very Low Density Lipoprotein
μM	Micro molar
BMI	Body Mass Index
CF	Cystic Fibrosis
HWE	Hardy-Weinberg Equilibrium
WBC	White Blood Cells
SPSS	Statistical Software for Social Sciences
OR	Odds Ratio
CI	Confidence Interval

Chapter 1

INTRODUCTION TO TROPICAL CHRONIC PANCREATITIS (TCP)

1.1. DEFINITION

Pancreatitis is a heterogeneous disease with varied etiologies, defined as an inflammatory disease of the pancreas leading to morphologic changes that typically cause pain and/or loss of function. Chronic pancreatitis (CP), [Online Mendelian inheritance in man (OMIM) 167800], is characterized by irreversible destruction and fibrosis of the exocrine parenchyma, leading to exocrine pancreatic insufficiency and progressive endocrine failure leading to diabetes. Histologic changes from the normal pancreatic architecture include irregular fibrosis, acinar cell loss, islet cell loss and inflammatory cell infiltrates, and distorted and blocked ducts [Kloppel et al. 1991]. Patients present at a young age with recurrent abdominal pain and diabetes and follow an accelerated course of the disease even with no history of alcoholism [Pitchumoni et al. 1984; Mohan et al. 1995]. According to Mitchell et al. [2003] in developed countries 60-70% of patients with CP have a long history of heavy alcohol consumption in male patients and unknown causes are responsible for 25% of cases, termed as idiopathic chronic pancreatitis (ICP). Tropical calcific pancreatitis (TCP, OMIM 608189) is a juvenile form of chronic calcific non alcoholic pancreatitis, seen almost exclusively in developing countries of the tropical world [Barman et al. 2003]. In the simplest terms, tropical calcific pancreatitis has been described as a disease with "pain in childhood, diabetes in puberty and death at the prime of life" [Geevarghese et al. 1985].

1.2. Demography of TCP in India and Elsewhere

The disease has most commonly been reported from Kerala but is prevalent throughout India. The prevalence of chronic pancreatitis in south India is very high and is estimated to affect 1 in 793, or 126/100000 in the population [Balaji et al. 1994], a figure far greater than the 10-15/100000, reported from the western countries and 45.4 per 100000 from Japan [Copenhagen Pancreatic Study Group 1981; Lin et al. 2000]. A recent population based study in southern India has shown the prevalence of TCP to be 0.02% in the general population [Mohan et al. 2008].

1.3. Etiology of CP

The etiology of TCP is unknown. Identified risk factors such as hypertriglyceridemia, hyperparathyroidism, obstruction of pancreatic duct by tumour, alcoholism and biliary stones are absent. It has been proposed that the consumption of cassava (Tapioca, Manilot esculents) or the protein energy diet may be the causative factor of the disease. But the disease may also affect the patients from higher economic background where malnutrition is unlikely.

1.4. Prevention and Cure

Unfortunately, very little is known about how to prevent or cure of this debilitating disease to date. For a long time, several genetic defects have been discovered to be associated with hereditary as well as idiopathic chronic pancreatitis in patients from Europe and United States. These studies have changed our understanding of the pathogenesis of CP. TCP resembles hereditary and idiopathic CP of Western countries in many clinical features. Genetic factors in the pathogenesis of pancreatitis were thought to be rare; recent progress in understanding the underlying causes came in 1996, when the genetic basis of the disorder was firmly established: Whitcomb and co-workers identified a germ line mutation in the gene encoding trypsinogen to associate with the disease phenotype [Whitcomb et al. 1996]. The finding of PRSS1 mutations causing HP and mutations in new genes (SPINK1 and CFTR) in patients with so-called idiopathic CP indicate that cases of CP with genetic risk factors in the background are much more common than originally envisioned. The expression of the cystic fibrosis transmembrane conductance regulator (CFTR) protein in pancreatic cells, its multiple functions and the presence of CFTR mutations in several disorders make the CFTR gene a potential candidate for involvement in pancreatitis. Biochemical investigations suggested that mutations in the cationic trypsinogen gene upset the protease antiprotease balance in the pancreas by promoting auto-activation of cationic trypsinogen to trypsin. Trypsin has the potential to activate the cascade of digestive enzymes prematurely within the pancreas, resulting in auto-digestion of the organ. Consistent with the central pathophysiological role of trypsin, loss-of-function alterations in the trypsin inhibitor gene predispose to various forms of pancreatitis by lowering the protective levels of the inhibitor. Recent data suggests that besides the "classic" autosomal dominant way of inheritance (HP), the autosomal recessive and multigenic inheritance pattern is also a common genetic background of the disease. Considerable effort has been directed toward understanding the mechanism of genetic abnormalities that predispose to CP; mutations of several candidate genes related to trypsinogen activation/inactivation are increasingly recognized for their potential disease-modifier role in distinct forms of CP. The above studies suggest that chronic pancreatitis irrespective of the etiology is possibly a multifactorial disease and occurs due to combination of the certain environmental factors and genetic predisposition. Therefore the present study is aimed to identify the role of interaction of multiple risk factors, gene-gene and gene-environment interaction in the development of tropical chronic pancreatitis.

Therefore the present work was taken up to find out and present the association of mutations in SPINK1 (N34S, IVS3+2T>C and IVS1-37T>C) and CFTR genes (ΔF508, G542X, G551D, R117H) S549N and IVS8-5T polymorphism. Also, we endeavoured to assess the association of mutations in Cathepsin B, ACE and MTHFR genes with TPC, if any, with the severity of CP in Indian population.

Chapter 2

LITERATURE SURVEY ON TROPICAL CHRONIC PANCREATITIS (TCP) RESEARCH

2.1. PANCREAS

In adult humans, the pancreas is a soft, elongated, flattened gland 12-20 cm in length and weighs about 80 g. Pancreas is a retroperitoneal organ and does not have a capsule. The second and third portions of the duodenum curve around the head of the pancreas. The spleen is adjacent to the pancreatic tail. The regions of the pancreas are the head, body, tail and uncinate process. The distal end of the common bile duct passes through the head of the pancreas and joins the pancreatic duct entering the duodenum. The functional unit of the exocrine pancreas is composed of an acinus and its draining ductule. The ductal system extends from the lumen of the acinus to the duodenum [Pandol et al. 2010]. A ductule from the acinus drains into interlobular (intercalated) ducts, which in turn drain into the main pancreatic ductal system. The acinus (from the Latin term meaning "berry in a cluster") can be spherical or tubular has some other irregular form (Figure 2.1). The acinar cells of the acinus are specialized to synthesize, store, and secrete digestive enzymes. Zymogens are flushed from the pancreas in a sodium bicarbonate rich fluid that is produced by the duct cells into the intestine, where they are activated. Activation of zymogens while they are still inside the pancreas can be highly destructive, so the exocrine pancreas incorporates redundant protective system to control the activity of these enzymes. If for any reason the protective system of the exocrine pancreas fails then it results in the activation of these zymogens within the pancreas which causes direct pancreatic injury resulting in pancreatitis. Pancreatitis is a heterogeneous disease of multifactorial etiology, which results in exocrine and endocrine insufficiency.

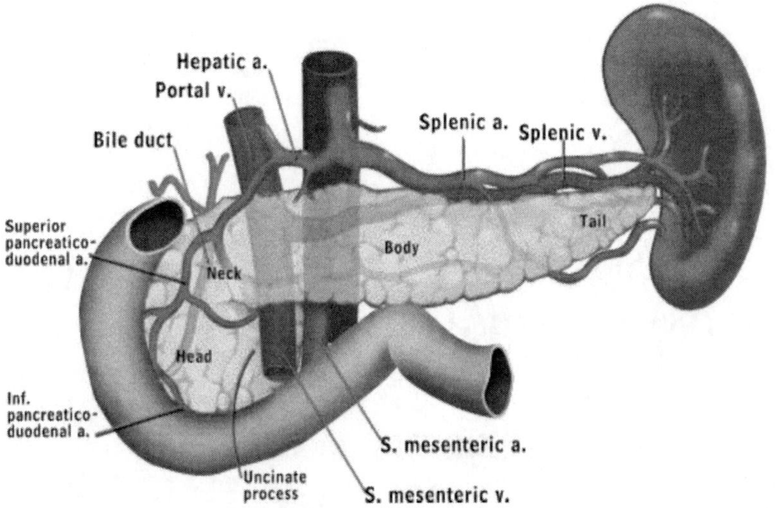

Structure of Pancreas

Figure 2.1. Adapted from Gorelick F, Pandol, SJ, Topazian M. Pancreatic physiology, pathophysiology, acute and chronic pancreatitis. Gastrointestinal Teaching Project, American Gastroenterological Association [2003].

2.2. Background Knowledge on Pancreatitis

In 1778 Cawley reported on a "free living young man" who had died of emaciation and diabetes and whose post-mortem examination revealed multiple pancreatic calculi [Mark et al. 1985]. Even, after the publication of various reports describing this disease, it still remains enigmatic. Dr. Chiari postulated that pancreatitis was caused by premature activated trypsin resulting in the auto-digestion of the pancreas [Chari et al. 1991].

Kini in 1937 described pancreatic calculi in an Indian patient for the first time. He operated on a 39 year old man with pancreatic calculi in 1937. The pancreas was hard and nodular, and the duct was dilated; external drainage was performed but the patient died on third day of operation. The term tropical pancreatitis (TP) was coined in 1955 when Zuidemia described 18 cases of disseminated pancreatic calcification in young non-alcoholic individuals in Indonesia [Zuidema et al. 1955; Zuidema et al. 1959]. These patients were diabetic and had marked emaciation resembling kwashiorkor. Zuidemia considered this entity to be a degenerative disease of the pancreatic parenchyma (pancreatic cirrhosis) secondary to protein malnutrition. The disease was characterized by younger age of onset, large intraductal calculi, exocrine and endocrine insufficiency and absence of other etiological factors.

In India it was first described by Geeverghese from the southern part of India and later on found to be prevalent in other parts also. The single largest series was described by Geeverghese and colleagues from the south-western state of Kerala in India where the disease was found to occur in endemic population. Geeverghese described the natural history of the disease as abdominal pain in childhood, diabetes in adolescence and death during the prime of life [Geeverghese et al. 1968].

Later on there was several reports of a similar syndrome from Asia (India, Ceylon, Thailand, Malaysia), Africa (Nigeria, Uganda, Burundi, Zaire, Malawi) and south America [Geeverghese et al.1962; Nagarathnam et al.1972; Kinnear 1963; Goodall et al.1964; Sonnet et al.1966; Olurin et al.1969; Dani et al.1976].

2.2.1. Definition

Chronic pancreatitis (CP) is usually recognised as disease with multifactorial etiology arising due to progressive destructive and inflammatory process of the pancreas, which may disturb its pathophysiological status. The primary characteristics of CP include irreversible obliteration of the endocrine and exocrine tissues which finally culminates into the clinical manifestation of CP [Whitcomb et al. 2004]. In certain tropical counties like India, a distinct etiology is not identified in a large number of chronic pancreatitis patients. Majority of these patients are young and the early-onset non-alcoholic form of idiopathic pancreatitis. In India such patients have been given a special name, viz., tropical chronic pancreatitis (TCP). Thus, tropical pancreatitis is a juvenile form of chronic calcific, non-alcoholic pancreatitis prevalent almost exclusively in the developing countries of the tropical world.

This form of CP has several unique characteristics that distinguish it from temperate zone pancreatitis: occurrence at young age, a more aggressive course to reach the end points of calculi formation, diabetes, steatorrhoea and pancreatic malignancy [Mohan et al. 1995; International Workshop on Types of Diabetes Peculiar to the Tropics 1996]. A subset of patients with TCP presents with diabetes without significant abdominal pain. This subset is also termed as Fibro calcific pancreatic diabetes (FCPD). Geeverghese described the natural history of the disease as abdominal pain in childhood, diabetes in adolescence and death during the prime of life [Expert Committee on the Diagnosis of Classification of Diabetes Mellitus 1997; Alberti et al. 1998].

2.2.2. Epidemiology of the Disease

The highest incidence of tropical pancreatitis in world appears to be in state of Kerala, India. Data from two large teaching hospitals in Kerala revealed that 12% to 16% of diabetic patients admitted had pancreatic calcification [Thomas et al. 1990]. An epidemiological study done in Kerala, showed that the prevalence of chronic pancreatitis in that community was 126/100 000 population and that of calcific pancreatitis was 98/100 000 population. These results were based on a study of 28567 healthy individuals belonging to 6079 families. The individuals were screened by a field study which included clinical examination, abdominal X- ray, pancreatic function test (benteromide test) and ultrasonography [Balaji et al. 1994; Copenhagen Pancreatic Study Group 1981]. The prevalence of CP in the Western world is about 10–15/100,000 population and in Japan about 45/100,000 population [Lin et al. 2000]. In a study from Madras showed that subjects with TCP have a significantly increased risk of pancreatic cancer [Chari et al. 1994]. In another study it has been shown that over 8 years of period 8.3% of the patients developed pancreatic cancer [Augustine et al. 1992]. The prevalence of FCPD (Fibrocalculous pancreatic diabetes) in south India constitute about 1% of diabetes patients seen at the M V Diabetes Specialities Centre, Chennai (formerly Madras), a large referral centre for diabetes in south India. Familial clustering of tropical pancreatitis has been reported, particularly in Kerala, raising the possibility of a familial or hereditary etiological factor. Family studies, however, did not reveal a specific pattern of inheritance [Pitchumoni et al. 1970].

2.3. Clinical Presentation of the Disease

Earlier reports suggested that patients were poor, extremely emaciated, young and emphasized the presence of protein-calorie malnutrition; bilateral parotid enlargement; distended abdomen and sometimes with a cyanotic hue of the lips [Geevarghese et al. 1968; Pitchumoni et al. 1984]. However recent report suggested that patients are diagnosed at an early age, usually between 15–30 years. A history of alcohol intake is absent. The most common presenting feature is recurrent severe abdominal pain, which is present in 80–90% of patients. Many patients have significant weight loss and vitamin deficiency. The patients develop insulin requiring diabetes but ketosis resistant below the age of 40 year's [Mittal et al. 2002]. Clinical features of TCP consist of triad: (1) Abdominal pain, (2) Diabetes and (3) Maldigestion leading to steatorrhoea.

2.3.1. Abdominal Pain

It is the predominant symptom and usually present in 30%-40% of patients. Pain is usually severe in upper abdominal position and radiating back [Pasricha et al. 2010; Raffaele et al. 2012]. Pain in the form of recurrent attacks of pancreatitis (signalling is not proper in exocytosis of acinar cell) the severity of pain decreases through progression of disease and it usually disappears with onset of exocrine insufficiency or diabetes. Pezzilli et al. (2007) said pain is the main symptom in CP and its treatment represents the main therapeutic option because pain severely impairs the quality of life.

2.3.2. Diabetes

Diabetes is an inevitable consequence of Tropical chronic pancreatitis (TCP) commonly occurring a decade or two after the first episode of abdominal pain. TCP is characterized as early pre-diabetic phase of the disease, while FCPD denotes syndrome of diabetes by World Health Organization [WHO study group report on diabetes mellitus 1985]. Fibrocalculous pancreatic diabetes (FCPD) is a form of diabetes, secondary to TCP seen in developing countries. In the majority of patients with TCP ultimately develop overt diabetes, in earlier stages of the disease, a stage of impaired glucose tolerance (IGT). There is a wide spectrum of patients treated with diet and oral agents. It is characterized by insulin requiring diabetes and presence of pancreatic calculi or other evidence of CP, e.g., dilated pancreatic ducts and mutations in the SPINK gene [Chandak et al. 2002].

2.3.3. Steatorrhoea/Maldigestion

Exocrine pancreatic insufficiency (EPI) and resultant maldigestion occur in up to 80% of patients following gastric, duodenal or pancreatic surgery. Patients with severe exocrine pancreatic insufficiency complain of passing bulky, frothy, or frankly oily stools. However, overt steatorrhoea is only present in about 20% of patients with TCP. The low frequency of steatorrhoea is attributed to the low fat intake in the diet [Barman et al. 2003]. When the fat intake of the diet was experimentally increased to 100 g/day from the average intake of 27 g/day, 76% of TCP patients developed steatorrhoea. Patients usually will present for evaluation when <10% of exocrine pancreatic function remains, which results in lipid malabsorption steatorrhea (frothy, foul smelling, buoyant stools), weight loss, abdominal discomfort, and abdominal swelling are the common presenting symptoms and are related to the inadequate lipid digestion [Ferrone et al. 2007; Layer et al. 2003]. Even with significant pancreatic insufficiency, protein and starch digestion are usually maintained at a normal physiologic level. However, once pancreatic insufficiency progresses, lipid malabsorption becomes the overriding problem and cause of many of the clinical symptoms and nutritional deficiencies. Abnormal lipid digestion leads to malnutrition, with malabsorption of lipid-soluble vitamins (A, D, E, and K), depleted micronutrients, and decreased circulating lipoproteins [Pezzilli et al. 2009].

2.4. Pathology

TCP is a progressive disease therefore the stages of pathogenesis depend on the specimen obtained.

2.4.1. Gross Pathology

The pancreas shows adhesions to the neighbouring organs. In humans on autopsy, the pancreas is usually found shrunken, hard due to fibrosis and ductal calculi. The parenchyma is often thin and atrophic and the pancreatic ducts are dilated with cystic spaces filled with stones [Pitchumoni et al. 1987]. It appears in dull white colour and the surface become irregularly nodular. The fibrosed zones are firm whereas the dilated ducts are soft and cystic. The stones can be easily palpated in the organ. In mild cases the size and appearance has been normal. The cut section of the pancreas shows the presence of homogenous areas with early to advanced fibrosis and intraductal calculi of varying shapes and sizes with marked dilation of the duct and ductules. Areas of dilation and stenosis may be seen in the same gland. The gland may get displaced from its normal location due to uneven shrinkage and fibrous adhesion. Calculi may vary in size, shape, and colour. Sections of calcified stones show epithelial debris, fibrin, and mucinous material. Colour of the stones varies from chalky white to dirty white [Barman et al. 2003].

2.4.2. Analysis of the Stones

Pancreatic calculi are composed of 95.5% calcium carbonate and small amount of calcium phosphate. The stones are initially soft and later enlarge and calcify; they are made of calcium carbonate (calcite) deposited on a protein lattice, and vary in size from small sand particles to calculi that are up to 20 g or more [Schultz et al. 1986]. Calculi have been found to have an amorphous nidus rich in iron, chromium, and nickel and a cryptocrystalline periphery containing a number of trace elements with a predominance of calcium.

2.4.3. Microscopy

The earliest changes are seen in acini which show patchy disruption, a characteristic feature of TCP. In later stages, diffuse fibrosis of the pancreas and ductal changes occur. While acini undergo regressive atrophic changes, ducts show proliferative and metaplastic changes, and often dilated and filled with mucus plugs. The characteristic cellular infiltration of the pancreas is composed of lymphocytes and plasma cells, distributed mainly around the ducts. Ductalization of acini also occurs in some cases. Dysplastic changes are seen in long standing cases. The most striking changes are found in the islets of Langerhans which show extensive nesidioblastosis, i.e. regeneration and formation of new islets [Nagalotimath et al. 1980; Nagalotimath et al. 1986].

2.4.4. Immunohistochemistry

Immunohistochemistry studies have shown paucity of alpha cells and beta cells. It shows a decrease in the number of islets in some cases and hyperplasia in others [Nair et al. 1994]. Nesidioblastosis may also be present in some patients (Figure 2.2). There is an overall decrease in the percent of insulin and glucagon cells. The decrease in insulin positivity in the islets often correlates with the serum Peptide levels and inversely with the duration of diabetes [Govindarajan et al. 2001].

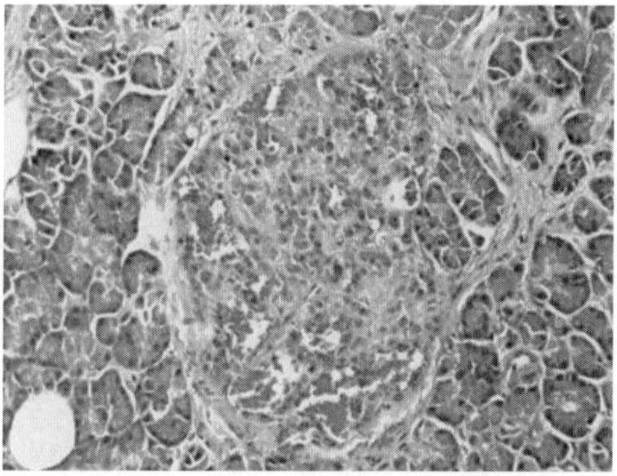

Figure 2.2. Histopathology showing Islet with prominent dilated capillaries which is associated with peliosis-like vascular ectasia. These findings were more common in patients with nesidioblastosis (Modern Pathology.2009; 22:239-245).

2.5. Diagnostic Tests for TCP

Diagnosis of pancreatitis is based on tests to assess structural and functional abnormalities which involve a collection of pancreatic secretions after intravenous administration of a secretagogue or a combination of secretagogue. The pancreas function tests can be divided into two categories: **(1)** the indirect tests of pancreatic function include measuring the released enzymes indirectly through its action on a substrate or its presence in stool or serum abnormality. **(2)** The direct tests of pancreatic secretory functions are summarised in Table 2.1.

Table 2.1. Laboratory tests used in the evaluation of the patients with suspected TCP

Test	Comments	References
Complete blood count	Elevated with infection, abscess	[Nair et al. 1994]
Serum amylase and lipase	Nonspecific for chronic pancreatitis	[Nagalotimath et al. 1986]
Total bilirubin, alkaline phosphatase, hepatic transaminase	Elevated in biliary pancreatitis and ductal obstruction by strictures or mass	[Nagalotimath et al. 1980]
Fasting serum glucose	Elevation suggests pancreatic diabetes	[Nair et al. 1994]
Pancreatic function tests	Sometimes useful in early chronic pancreatitis with normal computed tomography or magnetic resonance imaging	[Chase et al. 1996]
Fecal fat estimation	> 7 g fat per day is abnormal; quantitative; requires 72 hours; should be on a diet of 100 g fat per day	[Govindarajan et al. 2001]
Fecal elastase	< 200 mcg per g (0.20 g per kg) of stool is abnormal; non-invasive; exogenous pancreatic supplementation will not alter results; requires only 20 g of stool	[Chase et al. 1996]
Secretin stimulation	Peak bicarbonate concentration < 80 mEq per L (80 mmol per L) in duodenal secretion; best test for diagnosing pancreatic Insufficiency	[Seno et al. 1995; Ahmad et al. 2006]
Serum trypsinogen	< 20 ng per mL (0.83 nmol per L) is abnormal	[Govindarajan et al. 2001]
Lipid panel	Significantly elevated triglycerides are a rare cause of chronic pancreatitis	[Chase et al. 1996]
Calcium	Hyperparathyroidism is a rare cause of chronic pancreatitis	[Nair et al. 1994]
Immunoglobulin G4 serum antibody, antinuclear antibody, rheumatoid factor	Abnormality may indicate autoimmune pancreatitis	[Etemad et al. 2001]

2.6. Spectrum of Causes of Pancreatic Calcification

The discovery of pancreatic calcifications has long been used in the diagnosis of pancreatic disease, and for many years imaging of the pancreas was largely limited to the radiographic identification of these calcifications. Today, our ability to image the pancreas has greatly advanced with modalities including CT, sonography, endoscopic retrograde cholangiopancreatography, and MR imaging. This improved visualization of the pancreas allows better identification of pancreatic calcifications and their underlying causes. Pancreatic calcifications have been largely associated with chronic calcific pancreatitis from alcohol abuse. The entities that cause calcifications can help in an accurate diagnosis [Curry et al. 2000].

2.6.1. Pathological Tools for Assessments of Structural Abnormality in Pancreas during TCP

There are certain pathological techniques which are frequently used to assess the abnormal structural alterations in the human pancreas during CP. These are listed as following: (1) Plain Abdominal X-ray: Used to determine the pancreatic calcification, (2) Abdominal Ultrasonography: Most frequently used method for detecting the changes associated with CP. (3) Computed tomography (CT): The application of CT relates predominantly to the detection of complications. Besides the size and structure of the pancreas, the degree of ductal dilatation, calcification as well as the number and size of pseudocysts can be precisely assessed and showed in (Figure 2.3). (4) MRCP (Magnetic resonance cholangiopancreatography): MRCP permits native imaging of pancreatic ductal system. This is a useful non-invasive test; sensitivity is 70-80% as compared to ERCP. MRCP is able to provide high quality imaging of the pancreatic and biliary ducts in a noninvasive manner. (5) ERCP (Endoscopic retrograde cholangiopancreatography): ERCP has been thought to be the most specific and sensitive technique for the diagnosis of chronic pancreatitis [Bolan et al. 2003]. Ductal abnormalities detected using ERCP can be classified from normal to severe depending on the appearance of the main pancreatic duct, the number of abnormal ductal side branches identified, and the presence or absence of ductal obstruction, severe dilation, or irregularity. These criteria are taken together in Cambridge classification of pancreatographic findings of CP [Axon et al. 1984]. The sensitivity and specificity has been ranged from 70 - 90% and 80 -100%, respectively [Niederau et al. 1985; Forsmark et al. 2002; Bozkurt et al. 1994; Lankisch et al. 1995] (6) Endoscopic Ultrasonography (EUS): Endoscopic ultrasonography was developed in 1980s to perform high resolution imaging of the entire pancreas [Di Magno et al. 1980]. EUS can detect subtle parenchymal changes and minor ductal abnormalities in patients with CP by the use of high-frequency transducers [Wiersema et al. 1993; Kahl et al. 2002].

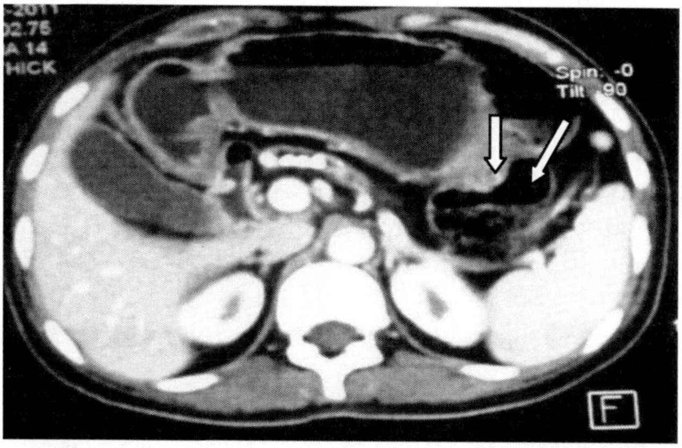

Figure 2.3. Contrast-enhanced CT scan shows small pancreatic calcifications (arrows) throughout gland. CT scan of patient conducted in our Institute; a case report.

2.7. Etiopathogenesis

The exact mechanism of pathogenesis remains an elusive. The following genetic and non-genetic factors have role in the disease development described in Table 2.2.

2.8. Environmental Factors

2.8.1. Role of Cassava and other Dietary Toxin

Cassava is a plant originating from South America and is known under various names: *Manihot esculenta*, manioc, yucca and tapioca. The tubers (part of the root system) and the leaves are used as food sources. It is an important staple in many developing countries of Africa, South and Central America, India and Southeast Asia. Since poverty and malnutrition were common in the countries from where the disease had been reported, malnutrition was suspected as a major causative factor and hence the disease was even described as “nutritional pancreatitis” [Millan et al. 1979]. Theoretically, excessive cassava consumption could lead to TCP in several ways. On ingestion, these may release hydrogen cyanide which is postulated to be toxic to the pancreas. It is in those regions of Kerala where cassava is the staple food that the highest prevalence of TCP has been noted. First, cassava is 87.5% carbohydrate with negligible (0.7%) protein content and essential amino acids (404 mg/100 g). Cassava contains the potentially toxic compounds, cyanogenic glycosides and consumption of cassava containing non-toxic levels of cyanide over long periods of time results in chronic cyanide toxicity. Cassava toxicity is also associated with malnutrition [Pitchumoni et al. 1988; Balakrishnan et al. 2006]. Aetiology parameters of CP in different countries are shown in Table 2.3.

Table 2.2. Aetiological risk factors for Tropical Chronic Pancreatitis

Environmental Cassava intake (cyanogenic glycosides)	Release HCN which may be toxic to pancreas; some epidemiological and experimental evidence
Oxidative Stress	Glutathione-S-transeferase (GST), MnSOD, Catalase, NADPH
Protein malnutrition	Severe deficiency causes pancreatic atrophy; unlikely to lead to CP
Genetic Serum protease inhibitor Kazal type 1 (SPINK1)	Specific pancreatic trypsin inhibitor, very strong association of p.N34S variant with TCP
Cystic fibrosis transmembrane regulator (CFTR)	Chloride channel, homozygous or compound heterozygous mutations cause cystic fibrosis
Cathepsin B	Lysosomal protease, association uncertain (only 1 report so far)
MTHFR	Methylene Tetrahydrofolate Reductase (only 1 report from Serbia on CP)
ACE	Angiotensin Converting Enzyme

Table 2.3. Aetiology of CP in different Countries according to a survey in the Asia Pacific Region (%)

Aetiology	Australia	China	India		Japan	Malaysia	South Korea	Singapore
			North	South				
Alcohol	95	18.8	41	25	54	35	70	39
Tropical	-	46.4	58	70	-	30	-	-
Idiopathic	5	25.1	-	-	35	30	26	61
Hereditary	-	5.6	-	-	0.17	5	0.8	-
Biliary	-	-	-	-	-	-	-	-
Others	-	9.7	1	5	11	-	3	-

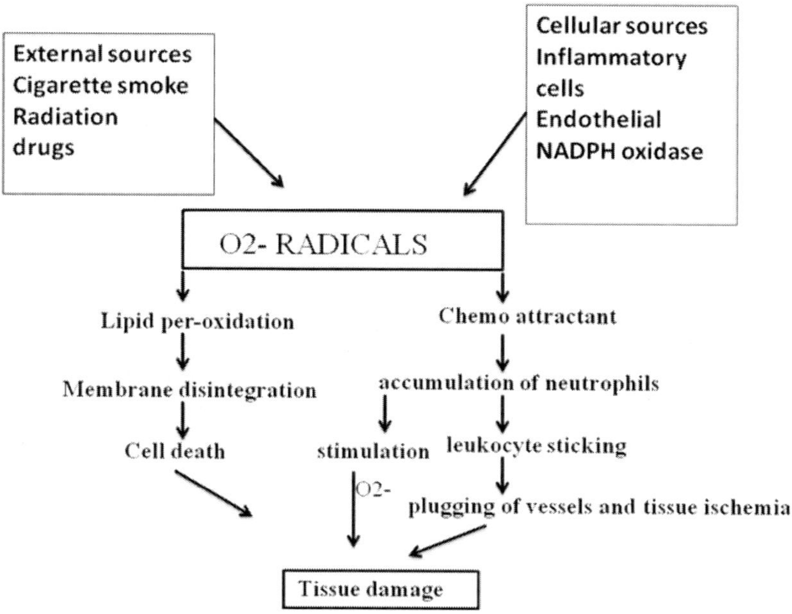

Source: Singh et al. (2013) Genetic and Environmental Attributes of Chronic Pancreatitis. British Journal of Applied Science and Technology 3(2):206-213.

Figure 2.4. Direct and indirect effects of oxygen free radicals.

2.8.2. Oxidative Stress in Pancreatic Inflammation

Reactive oxygen (ROS) and nitrogen species (RNS) have been implicated in the pathogenesis of CP. The electrophilicity of ROS/RNS make them highly susceptible to reaction with bio molecules including lipids, proteins and nucleic acid which alter the functionality of these molecules. The balance between ROS/RNS-generating enzymes and scavenger enzyme systems can be disrupted in a number of pathologic conditions, such as diabetes mellitus and pancreatitis, Switching on proinflammatory cascades not only exerts direct effects on the pancreatic cells, but also initiates the migration, adhesion, and infiltration of inflammatory cells into the exocrine pancreas [Kaneto et al. 2007; Singh et al. 2013]. These potentially harmful free radicals are scavenged by antioxidants. Many of these antioxidants are either essential nutrients or part of enzymes that maintain the critical balance between generation and destruction of free radicals. Deficiencies of antioxidants as observed in patients with both temperate and tropical pancreatitis led to the hypothesis that pancreatitis was caused by oxidative stress, defined as a state of potential tissue injury due to imbalance between injurious free radicals and protective antioxidants ROS can also disrupt mitochondrial membrane potential (øm), leading to cytochrome c release and subsequent DNA fragmentation [Ryter et al. 2007]. Such alternations in protein structure can affect enzyme activity, membrane-receptor function, and protein complex assembly. It is possible that several factors, including chronic induction of the cytochrome P450-1 subfamily of mono-oxygenase by xenobiotics (cigarettes, alcohol, occupational chemicals, dietary corn oil, and so forth) may be involved in the inflammation process [Apte et al. 2005]. The detailed mechanism is shown in Figure 2.4. However, the free radical hypothesis is by no means proven and certainly needs further studies.

2.9. Genetic Factors

A familial aggregation of the disease suggests a genetic aetiology. However, in contrast to hereditary pancreatitis, there is no definite mode of inheritance [Mohan et al. 1989]. The early age at onset and similarities with ICP, which has been shown to have a genetic basis, also suggest that similar genetic loci may be involved in its aetiology. Much of the recent advances in our knowledge of TCP have come from studies on the genetic aetiology of the disease in the past decade.

2.9.1. Genetics of Chronic Pancreatitis

More than 50 years ago, in 1952, it was reported that CP may cluster in selected families independent of additional environmental factors suggesting an inherited disease in these patients [Comfort et al. 1952]. The underlying genetic defect, however, remained obscure for more than 40 years. After genome-wide linkage analyses, three independent groups reported an association of the hereditary pancreatitis phenotype with the long arm of chromosome 7 in 1996 [Bodic et al. 1996; Pandya et al. 1996; Whitcomb et al. 1996a]. Within the same year the p.R122H mutation of the cationic trypsinogen gene was identified in all hereditary pancreatitis (HP) affected individuals and obligate carriers from five kindred' [Whitcomb et al. 1996b]. HP is an autosomal-dominant disorder with a clinical manifestation that is indistinguishable from other etiologic varieties of pancreatitis. The estimated penetrance of the disease is 70–80%. In affected patients, HP begins with recurrent attacks of acute pancreatitis that usually start in childhood or young adulthood. The attacks of pancreatitis frequently progress to chronic disease at an early age and are associated with a 40- to 50-fold increased lifetime risk for the development of pancreatic cancer [Lowenfels et al. 1997]. For a long time, genetic factors in the pathogenesis of pancreatitis were thought to be rare; however, the finding of PRSS1 mutations causing HP and mutations in new genes (SPINK1 and CFTR) in patients with so-called idiopathic CP indicate that cases of CP with genetic risk factors in the background are much more common than originally envisioned. Recent data suggests that besides the "classic" autosomal dominant way of inheritance (HP), the autosomal recessive and multigenic inheritance pattern is also a common genetic background of the disease. Considerable research effort has been directed toward understanding the mechanism of genetic abnormalities that predispose to CP; mutations of several candidate genes related to trypsinogen activation/inactivation are increasingly recognized for their potential disease-modifier role in distinct forms of CP [Teich et al. 2006]. The genetic loci known to predispose to CP includes SPINK1 (Serine Protease Inhibitor Kazal 1), CFTR (Cystic Fibrosis Transmembrane regulator).

2.9.2. Hereditary Pancreatitis

Trypsinogen is the most abundant digestive proteolytic pro-enzyme in the pancreatic juice. In humans it is secreted in three isoforms, cationic trypsinogen, anionic trypsinogen, and mesotrypsinogen encoded by the PRSS1, PRSS2 and PRSS3 genes, respectively. Cationic trypsinogen (~50–70%) and anionic trypsinogen (~30–40%) make up the bulk of trypsinogens in the pancreatic juice, while mesotrypsinogen accounts for 2–10%. The names have been designated according to the electrophoretic mobility of the proteins. Genetic variants of the gene encoding cationic trypsinogen (protease, serine 1; PRSS1) have been identified in patients with different forms of clinically idiopathic CP: hereditary pancreatitis (HP), familial pancreatitis or sporadic pancreatitis. The EUROPAC [European Registry of Hereditary Pancreatitis and Pancreatic Cancer] study states that the diagnosis of HP should be made on the basis of two first-degree relatives or three or more second degree relatives, in two or more generations with recurrent acute pancreatitis, and/or chronic pancreatitis for which there were no precipitating factors [Howe's et al. 2004]. Cases in which these strict criteria were not met, but more than one family member was carrying the disease, mostly within the same generation, are generally classified as familial chronic pancreatitis; the term sporadic refers to disease carriers with a negative family history.

The PRSS1 gene is about 3.6 kilobases long with five exons; more than 25 variants of the gene have been identified in patients with various forms of CP. Mutations are located in three clusters within the cationic trypsinogen sequence: in the trypsinogen activation peptide (TAP), in the N-terminal part of trypsin or in the longest peptide segment not stabilized by disulfide bridges between Cys64 and Cys139. Three PRSS1 mutations, namely R122H (~70%), p.N29I (~25%), and A16V (~4%), have been found with relatively high frequency in multiple families, whereas additional genetic variants have been identified only in very few patients [Teich et al. 2006]. The two most frequently occurring, thereby clinically relevant, R122H and N29I variants, which display a penetrance of 70–80%, are found exclusively in patients with a clear family history of pancreatitis, whereas p.A16V is a sporadic mutation, a genetic risk factor in CP [Witt et al. 1999]. Although many pedigrees have been reported, not all families described with clinically defined HP carry mutations in the PRSS1 gene. Consequently, the involvement of other yet unidentified genes may be significant in the disease pathogenesis. A familial aggregation of the disease suggests a genetic aetiology. However, in contrast to hereditary pancreatitis, there is no definite mode of inheritance. The genetic basis of the disease first reported that FCPD might share common susceptibility genes with type 1 and type 2diabetes. The molecular basis for hereditary pancreatitis has been attributed to mutations in exons 2 and 3 of the trypsinogen gene. Witt et al. showed that mutations in the SPINK1 gene are associated with chronic pancreatitis. Subsequently, exonic SPINK1 mutations, especially the N34S mutation, have been shown to be associated with idiopathic and chronic CP [Witt et al. 2000]. However, the incidence of this mutation is common, occurring in 0.5–2.5% of the general population. Since the studies on TCP and other form of CP have shown a strong association with SPINK1 gene, it is likely that this could be at least one of the predisposing factors to CP.

2.9.3. Serine Protease Inhibitor, Kazal Type 1 (SPINK1)

SPINK1, (OMIM 167790), also known as pancreatic secretory trypsin inhibitor, was first isolated from the bovine pancreas in 1948 [Kazal et al. 1948]. SPINK1 is synthesized by pancreatic acinar cells along with trypsinogen. The role of SPINK1 is the prevention of trypsin-catalyzed premature activation of zymogen within the acinar cells. SPINK1 can inhibit up to 20% of the tryptic activity in pancreas and is the first line of defence in protecting the pancreas against the autodigestion due to activation of trypsinogen to trypsin within the pancreas. Contrary to PRSS1 mutations which generate gain of function mutations; SPINK1 mutations cause a loss of function mutations, decreasing protease inhibition shown in Figure 2.5.

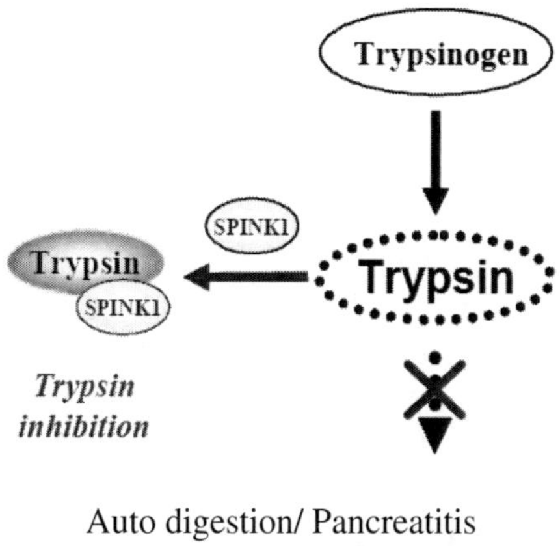

Figure 2.5. Trypsinogen a precursor form or zymogens' kept in pancreas and released in significant amount when needed for protein digestion, but when it is activated in pancreas itself then it leads to autodigestion of pancreas and inflammation. An inhibitor is present in pancreatic SPINK1 which binds to the active site of trypsin and inhibits the action of Trypsin.

The human SPINK1 gene is located on chromosome 5 and is comprised of approximately 7.1 kilobases, which contain four exons [Horii et al. 1987]. In 2000 Witt and co-workers screened the SPINK1 gene in 96 unrelated children and adolescents with idiopathic CP who did not have PRSS1 mutations and found mutation N34S in 23% of patients [Witt et al. 2000]. Data taken from eight larger studies in Europe and the United States indicate that 12.6% of patients with CP were heterozygous for N34S, and 3.6% were homozygous. Heterozygosity was detected at 1.9% in controls on average [Kiraly et al. 2007]. Thus the majority of carriers never develop pancreatitis, but the N34S mutation represents an important risk factor in CP. In addition to these studies, N34S was also recognized as a major genetic risk factor in tropical pancreatitis in the Indian subcontinent and as a minor susceptibility factor in alcoholic CP, in two diseases where PRSS1 mutations have no described role today. Taken together, the N34S alteration is considered to be a relatively frequent genetic susceptibility factor to CP, which exerts its effect in the context of other genetic and environmental factors, resulting in the highly variable penetrance and expression of the disease. Several other SPINK1 alterations have been described in recent years, mainly in single patients of families only (for detailed information of the different variants see [www.uni-leipzig.de/pancreasmutation].

2.9.4. N34S Variant

Subsequently, exonic SPINK1 mutations, especially the N34S mutation, have been shown to be associated with idiopathic and CP. However, the incidence of this mutation is common, occurring in 0.5–2.5% of the general population. By a candidate gene approach, SPINK1 was identified as another pancreatitis gene. In 18 out of 96 unrelated paediatric patients, a c.101A>G transition leading to substitution of asparagines by serine at codon 34 (N34S) was found. This variant was present in only 1 out of 279 control subjects (OR 62.2, P<1 10–10). Six patients were homozygous for this mutation [Witt et al. 2000]. N34S is mostly found in patients without a family history of CP, 15–40% of patients with so-called idiopathic CP carry N34S on one allele or on both alleles. Data taken from 8 larger studies in Europe and US showed that 12.6% of patients with CP were heterozygous for N34S, and 3.6% were homozygous [Witt et al. 2007]. The pathogenic mode of action of N34S, however, remains elusive. Recombinant N34S mutated human SPINK1 did not show any altered trypsin inhibitor capacity or secretion [Kiraly et al. 2007;

Boulling et al. 2007]. Patients with TCP display, in contrast to trypsinogen alterations, a very high incidence of SPINK1 variants, which is markedly more pronounced than that reported from Western countries. In 2002, four different research groups investigated Indian and Bangladeshi patients suffering from TCP, and all reported a strong association with the SPINK1 N34S alteration [Bhatia et al. 2000; Chandak et al. 2002; Hassan et al. 2002; Schneider et al. 2002]. Altogether, 351 patients and 973 control subjects were investigated in these studies. Approximately 9% of patients were homozygous for N34S and 29% heterozygous, compared to 0.2% and 4.3%in control individuals (Table 2.4).

Table 2.4. Frequencies of the SPINK1 N34S variant in TCP

Study	Patients				Controls			
	Number	Homozygous (%)	Heterozygous (%)	Wild-type (%)	Number	Homozygous (%)	Heterozygous (%)	Wild-type (%)
Chandak et al., 2002	68	11.8	33.8	54.4	100	0	3.0	97.0
Hassan et al., 2002	180	8.3	25.0	66.7	705	0.3	4.4	95.3
Bhatia et al., 2002	66	13.6	30.3	56.1	92	0	2.2	97.8
Schneider et al., 2002	37	2.7	37.8	59.5	76	0	1.3	98.7

2.9.5. IVS3+2T>C Variant

SPINK1 provides the first line of defence against prematurely activated trypsinogen by physically blocking the active site of trypsin. The IVS3+2T>C (c.194+2T>C) mutation is a loss- of –functional splicing mutation; it affects the consensus splicing donor site in intron 3 and may cause skipping of the entire exon 3, where the trypsin-binding site is located. In our study we found N34S (heterozygous) mutation in 10 (6.7%) cases and 1 (0.67%) in controls which shows significant association of IVS3+2T>C mutation with chronic pancreatitis risk (OR: 10.6, 95%CI: 1.34-84.26, p-value: 0.014). A sole report of mutated SPINK1 in a TCP patient outside the Indian subcontinent exists [Snabbon et al. 2006].

2.9.6. IVS1-37T>C Variant

The IVS1-37T>C and c.101A>G (N34S) variants occurred together in one family without trypsinogen mutations and were present in the same haplotype. They have been classified as neutral polymorphisms based primarily on the fact that they did not segregate with the disease and that they were present in control chromosomes. *Thread Gold* showed that [N34S; IVS1–37T-C] mutation was associated with familial, idiopathic, and autoimmune CP. Three of 8 (38%) patients with familial pancreatitis had the N34S mutation, in agreement with the previous report showing a strong association between N34S mutation and familial pancreatitis. N34S; IVS1–37T 1 C mutation in 4 of 31 patients with idiopathic CP. Thus, 7 of 39 (18%) patients with familial or idiopathic CP carried this mutation.

2.9.7. Cystic Fibrosis Transmembrane Conductance Regulator Gene (CFTR)

Cystic fibrosis (CF), the most common life-shortening autosomal recessive disease in Caucasians, is classically described as a triad of chronic obstructive pulmonary disease, exocrine pancreatic insufficiency and elevation of sodium and chloride concentration in the sweat. CF is caused by loss-of-function mutations in CFTR, which encodes a cAMP-activated chloride channel in epithelial cell membranes and regulates other membrane transport proteins [Whitcomb et al. 2010].

F508del is the most common CF-causing mutation. F508del homozygous generally has <2% of normal CFTR function and typically have pancreatic insufficiency. In contrast, CF patients with genotypes producing ~5% of normal CFTR function often have pancreatic sufficiency. Genotypes with even higher residual CFTR function (~10% of normal) are associated with congenital bilateral absence of the vas deferens (CBAVD), a disease causing infertility in males who have normal pulmonary, pancreatic, and sweat gland function. In these cases, the genotypes consist of a severe mutation plus a mild mutation that reduces CFTR function 10~30% of normal [Cohn et al. 2005]. In 1998, Sharer and colleagues and Cohn and colleagues were able to show an association of CFTR mutations with chronic pancreatitis [Sharer et al. 1998; Cohn et al. 1998]. The variety of pancreatic disorders in cystic fibrosis ranges from complete loss of exocrine and endocrine function to almost normal pancreatic function. Recently published studies confirmed the association of

CP and CFTR mutations, but until now the underlying mechanisms leading to the development of CP are inadequate.

Riordan and colleagues in Toronto first cloned the CFTR gene in 1989. It is a 250 kb gene located on long arm of chromosome 7 encoding 1480 amino acids polypeptide, named cystic fibrosis transmembrane conductance regulator (CFTR), which function as a chloride channel in epithelial membrane [Riordan et al. 1989]. The nucleotide sequence was translated into the primary amino acid sequence to reveal a protein with 1480 amino acids The amino acid sequence was found to be homologous to nucleotide (ATP)-binding folds (NBFs) in two places. Additionally, there were two sets of six hydrophobic regions capable of spanning the lipid bilayer of the cell membrane, thus embedding the protein in the membrane. Lastly, between the two NBFs was a highly charged regulatory (R) domain that showed similarity to sequences for phosphorylation by protein kinases A or C (PKA and PKC) [Fanen et al. 2011]. While most ABC transporters consist of four domains (two membrane-spanning and two nucleotide-binding domains), CFTR is the only one known to possess a regulatory domain. Modification of the regulatory domain, either through the addition or removal of chemical phosphate groups, has been shown to regulate the movement of chloride ions across the membrane [Gadsby et al. 2006]. The CFTR gene and its exonic and intronic sequences are shown in Figure 2.6.

Over 1000 mutations and polymorphisms of the CFTR gene have been reported since its identification in 1989 [Riordan J et al. 1989]. The most frequent mutation in the CFTR gene is delta F508 mutation (deletion of three base-pair which results in omission of phenylalanine) located on exon 10 and is identified in nearly 70% of patients with cystic fibrosis [Kabra et al. 2003]. The CFTR genotype (severe or moderate mutations) depends on the expression of the functional CFTR protein and controls phenotype severity (lung disease, pancreatic insufficiency, agenesis of the vas deferens) [Tsui et al. 2001].

CFTR conducts both chloride and bicarbonate and is essential for normal bicarbonate secretion by pancreatic duct cells, which have the function of a protective mechanism centering on flushing and draining secretion, because the luminal concentrations of calcium is relatively high and the protection of the pancreas by autolysis of trypsin at R122 is no longer possible [Cohn et al. 1998].

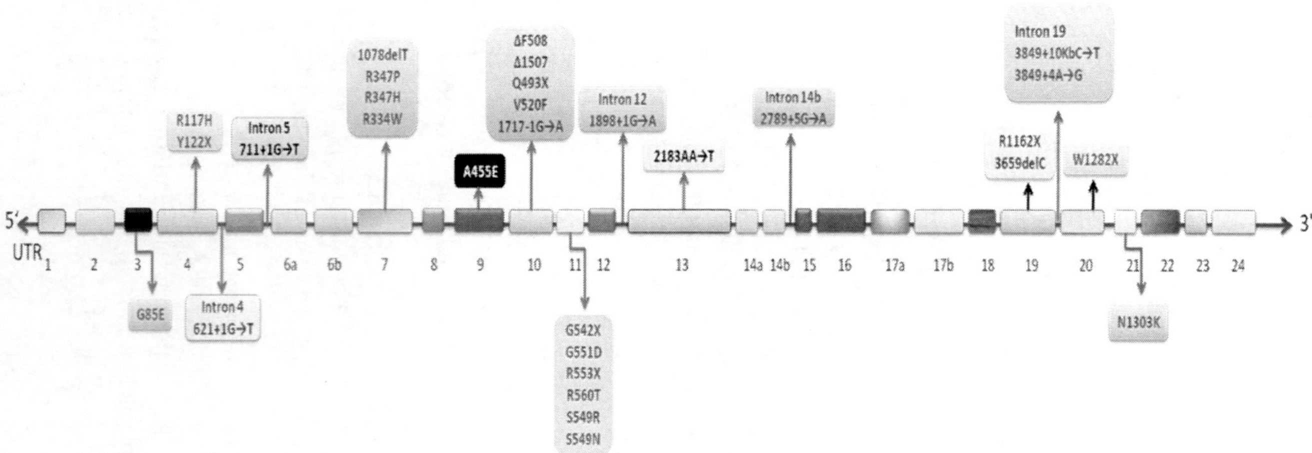

Figure 2.6. CFTR gene and its exonic and intronic sequences.

More than 1200 CFTR gene polymorphism have been reported which can be divided into six classes, based on the functional consequences of the polymorphism on the channel function:

Class I –III mutations are severe ($CFTR^{sev}$)
Class I mutations: defective protein synthesis
Class II mutations: abnormal processing trafficking
Class III mutations: defective activation and all result in functional loss of CFTR from the epithelial cell surface
Class IV mutations: mild variable mutations ($CFTR^{m-v}$) and all result in reduction but not absence of channel ion conductance
Class V mutations: diminish protein synthesis or stability
Class VI mutations: may affect the regulatory function of CFTR on other ion channels

The increased frequency of CFTR mutations has been reported in up to 30% of patients with idiopathic chronic pancreatitis [Marie et al. 2003]. The frequency of CFTR mutation in these patients was six times higher than expected, whereas the frequency of the 5T allele was twice as high. Also, the frequency of CFTR mutation in alcohol related pancreatitis was two times higher than expected [Perri et al. 2003].

Some of these mutations involve a single allele, whereas others are a combination of a severe and a mild mutation or either type of mutation with the 5T allele in intron 8, which reduces the amount of functional CFTR [Maltas et al. 2001].

There are several distinct situations

1. The most severe genetic risk is associated with $CFTR^{sev}/CFTR^{sev}$ genotype, which determines typical cystic fibrosis and the pancreas histology, includes all of the features of the chronic pancreatitis.
2. Patients with genotype $CFTR^{sev}/CFTR^{m-v}$ develop atypical cystic fibrosis having a residual CFTR function (less than 10 % of normal); these patients are at increased risk of pancreatitis (approximately 80%), but most of them do not develop the disease Recurrent acute pancreatitis and chronic pancreatitis occurs in the context of other environmental or genetic risk factors.
3. A distinct category is the presence of heterozygous CFTR mutations, which increases the risk of recurrent acute and chronic pancreatitis. In this category there are also three possible situations:

a. Patients with CFTR $^{m\text{-}v}$/ CFTR $^{m\text{-}v}$ genotype and atypical cystic fibrosis, associated with mutations that are not included in cystic fibrosis screening panels, which increase the risk of pancreatic injury. These specific mutations appear to disrupt the function of exon 9 and 10 of the CFTR gene product
b. Patients with a complex disorder such as polygenic CFTR-SPINK1 pancreatitis, with heterozygous CFTR and heterozygous SPINK1 mutations occurring together
c. Patients with some specific CFTR variants which may increase the susceptibility to environmental factors, especially to alcohol [Casals et al. 2004].

Data on CFTR variants in CP are very limited and so far only a single study exists. Although all 27 CFTR coding exons, including the 5T allele, were analysed, the study population consisted of only 18 Indian TCP patients [Bhatia et al. 2000]. Two patients (11%) showed a CFTR variant: one subject was homozygous for 5T and the other heterozygous for p.R1070Q, which is presumed to be a mild missense variant. The overall frequency of CFTR alterations was 0.083 (3/36), which was far lower than that observed in white Caucasian subjects with CP (0.20–0.24). One study tested 411 patients with CP, 242 had idiopathic aetiology, nine patients had mutation and 41 patients had polymorphism ($p<0.001$) [Midha et al. 2010]. Subsequent studies analyzing the complete CFTR coding sequence as well as PRSS1 and SPINK1 found that in Western countries 25% to 30% carried at least one CFTR mutation, but only few patients were compound heterozygous [Audrézet et al. 2002]. CF mutation plus a milder allele in trans causes increased risk of idiopathic pancreatitis, severe allele comprising a milder allele [Lebo et al. 2007]. In our study, we have described a case of alcoholic chronic pancreatitis with hemoglobinopathy, the patient was found compound heterozygous for SPINK1 gene mutation [N34S and IVS3+2(T-C)] and heterozygous for CFTR gene [G551D/N] [Singh et al. 2013]. Further genetic studies are necessary to elucidate the significance of CFTR variants in TCP.

2.9.8. Cathepsin B

The lysosomal cysteine protease cathepsin B (CTSB), (OMIM 116810) is presumed to perform an essential role in the intrapancreatic activation of digestive enzymes by mediating premature trypsinogen activation [Gorelick et al. 1995]. The mechanism responsible for the intrapancreatic activation of digestive zymogens is unknown, but a recent hypothesis predicts that a redistribution of lysosomal cathepsin B (CTSB) into a zymogen-containing subcellular compartment triggers this event [Figarella et al. 1988]. Moreover, after induction of experimental caerulein-induced pancreatitis, Ctsb knock-out mice displayed a lowered trypsin activity within the gland and a diminished acinar necrosis compared to wild-type animals [Halangk et al. 2000]. To test the cathepsin B hypothesis more directly and to overcome the shortcomings of lysosomal enzyme inhibitors, which have only limited specificity for CTSB, we have used a CTSB-deficient mouse strain that was generated by targeted disruption of the ctsb gene [Deussing et al. 1998]. Recently, *Mahurkar and co-workers* performed a mutational analysis of CTSB and found an association between TCP and a c.76C>G transversion in exon 3, leading to leucine by valine exchange at codon 26 (L26V) [Mahurkar et al. 2006]. Investigating 306 Indian patients with TCP and 330 controls, the 26V allele was significantly overrepresented in patients (minor allele frequency 0.46) compared to control subjects (minor allele frequency 0.29) with P-0.013. According to our own preliminary investigation among patients from north India, we found 150 patients with TCP and 150 control subjects with L26V odds ratio (OR) of 1.9 (95% confidence interval (CI) 1.50–2.50, (p value = 0.03) (unpublished data).

2.9.9. Methylenetetrahydrofolate Reductase (MTHFR)

The pancreas contains high level of folate, second only to the liver as evidenced from experimental studies which proved an association between folate levels and pancreatic disease [Balaghi et al. 1993]. Some studies have suggested that reduced exocrine function was a result of disturbed methyl metabolism secondary to folate deficiency [Parsa et al. 1972]. It is possible that the disturbed metabolism may cause abnormal cellular differentiation, reduced exocrine function of the pancreas, increased toxic injury and carcinogenesis as a consequence of autolytic destruction of the pancreas in chronic pancreatitis, which has been associated with pancreatic cancer [Donghui et al. 2005]. Chronic inflammation in pancreatitis induces DNA damage and mutations and thereby facilitates the development of pancreatic cancer. The processes like DNA synthesis during replication and repair are largely dependent on the availability of one carbon metabolism pathway. Therefore, one-carbon metabolism polymorphisms may have the potential to modify or influence chronic pancreatitis [Suzuki et al. 2008].

The MTHFR gene contains a 2.0-kbp coding region with 11 exons and is located on chromosome 1p 36.3. It is a key enzyme in folate metabolism that catalyzes the conversion of 5, 10- methylenetetrahydrofolate (5, 10- methylene THF) to 5-methyltetrahydrofolate (5-methyl THF,) a predominant circulatory form of folate and methyl donor for the remethylation of homocysteine to methionine [Fodinger et al. 2000]. Methionine is the principal methyl donor for the methylation process. A reduction in MTHFR activity such as that caused by the C to T transition at position 677 of the MTHFR cDNA (C667T) or change in the alanine to valine at position 222 of the MTHFR amino acid sequence, produces a thermolabile enzyme which results in increased plasma homocysteine level [Hai-Xia et al. 2008; Ivan et al. 2008]. There were many reports of MTHFR with developmental disorders like neural tube defects (such as spina bifida, nonsyndromic cleft lip and Down's syndrome) and neurological impairment [Vander et al. 1998; Hobbs et al. 2000; Song et al. 2001; Miao et al. 2002]. Though there is a worldwide distribution of a common MTHFR mutation, previous studies of C667T mutation mainly concentrated on European population [Schneider et al. 1998]. In our study conducted on North Indian population showed the frequency of the MTHFR was 57.3%, 34.1% and 8.5% among cases compared with 87.2%,11.2% and 1.5% of controls for CC, CT and TT genotypes, respectively. The T Allele frequency was found significantly higher in patients than in controls. A significant association with T allele was observed with p-value <0.0001, odds ratio 4.475 and 95% CI=2.961-7.046. Since, numerous environmental factors play important role in the etiologies of chronic pancreatitis, therefore, in our study we have observed a clear dose-response relationship in the interaction between cigarette smoking and MTHFR 677 TT genotype in the study population with OR 4.139(95% CI=2.23-7.673) and (P<0.001) [Singh et al. 2012; Talamini et al. 1999]. The results of one study published so far by Ivan and Jelena [Ivan et al 2008] have indicated increased frequency (51%) of the C677T polymorphism in CP patients in Serbian population but it was not statistically significant with P-0.458.

2.9.10. Angiotensin Converting Enzyme

The renin-angiotensin system (RAS) is a circulatory cascade system primarily involved in the regulation of blood pressure and serum electrolytes [Peach et al. 1977; Stroth et al. 1999]. Correlations between hypertension and diabetes mellitus have become the basis to examine rennin-angiotensin system

(RAS) in the pancreas. The RAS participates in the development of inflammation and fibrosis in the heart, kidney, lung and liver through the regulation of cell growth and inflammation, induction of oxidative stress and worsening of fibrosis. They are mainly executed by angiotensin II, the product of hydrolysis of angiotensin I by angiotensin-converting enzyme (ACE) [Leung et al. 2003]. The activities of ACE and RAS are known to be enhanced during acute pancreatitis and chronic hypoxia in experimental animals. All components of RAS are intrinsically present in the pancreas, and the level of RAS is enhanced in animal models of pancreatic diseases suggesting a role for RAS in the development of pancreatitis. The inhibition of RAS with ACE inhibitors and Angiotensin II Receptor Blockers (ARB) was reported mostly to ameliorate the development of acute and chronic pancreatitis in rat models, Wistar Bonn/Kobri rats [Barbara et al. 2010]. A frequent ACE insertion/deletion (I/D) alteration in intron 16 exists that accounts for nearly half of the variation of serum ACE levels [Rigat et al. 1990]. A study investigated the ACE I/D variant in 171 Indian subjects with TCP and compared the genotype and allele frequencies with 99 ethnically matched healthy controls [Bhaskar et al. 2006]. No significant differences with TCP per se, as well as with fibrosis or progression of the disease, were observed. The authors concluded that the ACE I/D variant do not play a role in the pathogenesis of TCP. In other study conducted by Nevin Oruc in 79 patients' no association was reported [Nevin et al. 2009]. ACE gene I and D allele frequency of patients (44% and 56%) were similar to controls (45% and 55%). There were no significant differences in severity of pancreatitis between patients with the ACE-insertion or ACE-insertion/deletion versus ACE-deletion genotypes. No significant difference was observed in clinical features between patients with ACE-insertion or insertion/deletion genotypes vs. patients with ACE-deletion genotype in sporadic and familial pancreatitis [Nevin et al. 2004]. Our unpublished data showed the allele frequency of the ACE deletion was 55.3% in CP patients and 53.1% in healthy controls (odds ratio-1.09, 95% CI 0.825-1.434, P - 0.5845). Frequency of the ACE-DD genotype was 28% as compared to the II and ID genotypes was found 38.7% and 33.7% as compared to control 30.7%, 37.1% and 32.2% with no significant difference p-0.835.

2.9.11. Gene-Gene Interaction in Chronic Pancreatitis

A further complexity exists in the phenomena of genotype-phenotype correlation in gene-gene interaction. PRSS1 gain of function mutation, with the exception of A16V, was found predominantly in patients with HP and FCP [Rossi et al. 1998]. We conclude that there was a very small additional risk conferred by the N34S allele, and it has been completely compromised by PRSS1 R122H mutation. There is a low-penetrance with N34S allele. A pilot study from Bangladesh on 11 FCPD and five chronic calcific pancreatitis patients without diabetes mellitus reported lack of R117H mutation in the PRSS1 gene [Chandak et al. 2002]. Analysis of the phenotype in terms of the age of onset, frequency of attacks, and presence and age of onset of diabetes mellitus did not show any significant difference between N34S heterozygous or homozygous patients. But SPINK1 N34S when co inherited with the low-penetrance PRSS1A16V may contribute to the phenotypic expression of ICP [Weiss et al. 2003].

Gene-gene interaction has been documented when individuals who inherited both low penetrance SPINK1 variations along with CFTR mutation in ICP may. Coinheritance of N34S allele and an abnormal CFTR allele accounts for 4% (1/25), 5.1% (2/39) of the total patients analyzed and the diagnosis of CP was unambiguous [Noone et al. 2001; Tzetis et al. 2007]. So a synergistic effect was observed between compound heterozygote CFTR allele and the SPINK1 N34S allele. The risk of pancreatitis is increased by ~40 fold by having two CFTR mutations, 20 fold by having N34S and 900 fold by having both [Noone et al. 2001]. So it likely confers an additive or a multiplicative effect between two genes which are involved in a common pathway. Different pathway genes also confirm the risk but it may take long progression of disease.

2.9.12. Genetic Implication in Diagnosis

Diagnosing CP, especially just after the onset of the disease, is a very difficult task. The diagnosis is often made only several years after the first pancreatitis attack when functional and structural abnormalities of the pancreas surface and are detected with laboratory studies and imaging. But what about genetic testing ? Until now genetic testing in CP patients is not part of any standard diagnostic procedure, with the possible exception of PRSS1 mutations in HCP cases [Monique et al. 2010]. The presence of a genetic mutation provides more insight in the cause of the disease. This is important for caregivers, but also for patients, who are often hold culpable of alcohol abuse. Genetic testing, however, raises questions: Do all reported genes need to be tested or only those with the highest association? What to do if the mutation is found? Should we screen the whole family members? Does a mutation change anything to the prognosis or management of the disease?

Genetic testing for all the genes associated with pancreatitis is advisable; including testing for SPINK1 mutation, which should be approved by Research Ethics Committee. This should be followed by counselling. If a mutation is found in the patient then it should be kept in mind that patients need not to worry about the management and inheritance of mutation. He should be guided that mutation does not affect clinical course of disease and the management. One should be advised about the lifestyle as it affects the course of the disease. Tobacco and smoking increase the progression of the disease and finally leads to pancreatic cancer [Lowenfels et al. 2001].

2.9.13. Treatment and Management

Conservative treatment goals of uncomplicated CP are pain control, relief of mechanical obstruction or complications, correction of malabsorption and diabetes. Pancreatic extracts are frequently administered to improve absorption and reduce pain. Cessation of alcohol ingestion is essential because the 5-year mortality rate of chronic pancreatitis in patients who continue to abuse alcohol is 50 percent [Mergener et al. 1997]. If pain is increasing or intractable, imaging should be performed to assess for complications such as pseudocyst or mechanical obstruction. Surgery, either open or endoscopic, can be helpful in such cases. The attractive feature of endoscopic procedures is that they offer an alternative to surgery. The goal of endoscopic treatment for chronic painful pancreatitis with pancreatic duct stones is clearance of calculi from the duct, thus relieving the obstruction and pain. [Adler et al. 2006]. Celiac plexus nerve block is performed frequently for long-term pain control. Unfortunately, no causal treatment of TCP is known today. In patients monitored for more than 10 years, the mortality rate is 22% and pancreatitis induced complications account for 13% of the deaths. The causes of death are alcoholic liver disease, postoperative complications, and cancer. Older age at diagnosis, cigarette smoking, and alcohol intake are major predictors of mortality among individuals with chronic pancreatitis [Chari et al. 1994]. The risk of developing pancreatic cancer is significantly higher in patients with CP than in the general population. Alcoholic CP and tropical pancreatitis are associated with a 15-fold and a 5-fold increased risk of pancreatic cancer, respectively [Steer et al. 1995], whereas the cumulative lifetime risk of cancer in patients with hereditary pancreatitis is reported to be as high as 40%. Mortality in CP, particularly alcoholic, is approximately one-third higher compared to an age- and sex-matched general population [Lowenfels et al. 2005].

CP is a unique form of CTP seen exclusively in some tropical countries of the world. The prognosis of TCP patients has improved in the last two to three decades and the understanding of the natural history of TCP. The higher prevalence of TCP in the Indian subcontinent, in comparison to ICP in the West, as well as areas of endemicity, still needs to be explained. More frequent detection of PRSS1, SPINK1 and CFTR defects in pancreatitis patients than in the general population opened a new chapter in diagnostics of idiopathic pancreatitis and understanding of molecular mechanisms of the disease. It is to be expected that future CP genes will have less effect on the phenotype, and will be associated with less than 5% of the set of CP cases. The biggest challenge is to find the candidate genes that are responsible for ACP, the most common form of CP, and the quest for genetic etiological factors is ongoing. Whether this is due to differences in genetic predisposition, specific environmental factors, or, as is most likely, a combination of both, still needs to be ascertained. Further studies should explore the pathogenesis mechanism that could pave the way for prevention of the disease. Underlying genetic variants are central CP susceptibility and progression. Three genes, with Mendel genetic biology (PRSS1, CFTR and SPINK1) have been recognized for over a decade, and little progress has been made since then. Furthermore, application of high-throughput genetic techniques including genome-wide association studies (GWAS) and next generation sequencing (NGS) will provide a large volume of new genetic variants associated with CP, but with small independent effect that are impossible to apply in the clinic. The problem of interpretation is using the old framework of the germ theory of disease to understand complex genetic disorders. A new frame work based on modelling and simulation of physiological processes with or without genetic, metabolic and environmental variables considered at the cellular and organ levels, with integration of the immune system, nervous system, tissue injury and repair system, and DNA repair system. The effort is needed to target the etiology of pancreatic dysfunction beginning at the first signs of disease and there by prevent the development of irreversible damage and complication of TCP.

Chapter 3

MAIN OBJECTIVES OF THE STUDY ON TROPICAL CHRONIC PANCREATITIS

1. To assess the type and frequency of CFTR and SPINK1 gene mutation and polymorphism in cases with tropical chronic pancreatitis (TCP) and controls in North Indian patients.
2. To investigate the genetic polymorphisms of CTSB gene mutation and its association with severity of disease.
3. To investigate the genetic polymorphisms of MTHFR and ACE gene polymorphism and its association with TCP
4. To establish a genotypic and phenotypic correlation
5. Extended family screening to check the inheritance pattern.

Chapter 4

EXPERIMENTAL DESIGN AND PROCEDURES USED IN STUDY OF TROPICAL CHRONIC PANCREATITIS

4.1. STUDY DESIGN AND SETTING

This was a hospital based case-control study jointly conducted at Department of Medical Genetics and Department of Gastroenterology, Sanjay Gandhi Post Graduate Institute of Medical Sciences (SGPGIMS), Lucknow, Uttar Pradesh, a tertiary care center in Northern India from October 2009 to 2012.

4.2. SUBJECTS AND METHOD

4.2.1. Subjects

All consecutive patients in three years of time with TCP attending the Gastroenterology O.P.D. at S.G.P.G.I.M.S. Lucknow were included in the study as per inclusion criteria. Clinical diagnosis was based on phenotype and radiological criteria and exocrine function tests. Patients giving the history of occasional alcohol consumption were excluded from the study.

Subjects	Total number
Tropical Chronic Pancreatitis	150
Healthy control	150

4.2.1.1. Diagnosis: Inclusion Criteria for TCP

1. Radiological evidence of pancreatic intraductal calcification
2. Non-alcoholic
3. No family history of Pancreatitis

4.2.1.2. Exclusion Criteria for TCP

1. Absence of any other etiological factor like alcoholism, hypercalcaemia, gall stones
2. Presence of pancreatic cancer

4.2.1.3. Inclusion Criteria for Control

1. Age and Sex matched control
2. No history of Pancreatitis.
3. Absence of any other cause for abdominal pain

4.2.1.4. Exclusion Criteria for Control

1. Presence of pancreatic cancer
2. History of alcohol ingestion

4.2.1.5. Sample Size Calculation

Sample size was estimated on the basis of previously published data using QUANTO software (version 1.2.3) for each genetic polymorphism. We have made the assumptions of matched case-control study considering 80% power and ≤0.05 level of significance

4.3. Molecular Analysis

4.3.1. DNA Extraction from Whole Blood

2 ml of blood sample in EDTA vial was collected separately from all the patients and age and sex matched controls. Samples were stored at -80C for further analysis. DNA extraction was done by standard phenol-chloroform method described by Ponez et al. (1982) with minor modifications. The following steps were used.

4.3.2. Lysis of Red Blood Cells

To the whole blood (2 ml), RBC lysis solution (NH_4Cl 7 g/lit and NH_4HCO_3 0.072 g/lit) was added and mixed thoroughly by inverting the tubes several time. The tubes were then centrifuged at 2500rpm at 4^0C for 10 min, the supernatant was discarded. This procedure was repeated until the pellet becomes colourless. This pellet is enriched with WBCs.

4.3.3. Lysis of White Blood Cells

The WBC pellet was suspended in 4 ml of STE solution [0.05 M NaCl, 0.01 M Tris Buffer and 0.007M EDTA pH (6.5)]. To this 200μl of 10% SDS and 20 μl of (100 μg/ml) of proteinase K was added. The tubes were kept for overnight incubation at 37ºC in an incubator. Complete lysis of WBC was judged by progressive increases of viscosity of the solution.

4.3.4. Phenol-Chloroform Extraction

An equal volume of Tris saturated phenol [200mM Tris buffer (pH8.0), 0.01% Hydroxyquinoline] was added to the WBC lysate mixed well and allow stand for 10 min at 4^0C then centrifuged at 2500 rpm at 4^0C for 10 minutes. The aqueous phase was recovered for further use. To this an equal volume of a mixture of chloroform: isoamyl alcohol (24:1v/v) and tris saturated phenol was added and allowed to stand at 4^0C for 10 minutes and centrifuged at 2500 rpm at 4^0C for 10 minutes. The aqueous phase was recovered for precipitation of DNA.

4.3.5. Precipitation of DNA

To the aqueous phase, approximately 5 volume of chilled absolute ethanol was added. As ethanol was being added DNA fibers solve out of the solution and become visible to the naked eye. The DNA was recovered by centrifugation at 2500 rpm at 4^0C for 10 minutes. The tubes were kept for 1-2 hours at 4^0C for complete precipitation of the DNA. The precipitated DNA was separated and air-dried and was dissolved in 200 μl of HPLC grade water.

The high molecular weight DNA was allowed to dissolve completely by keeping it at 37^0C for a night.

4.3.6. Quality and Quantity Assessment of DNA

The quality of the DNA was checked on 0.8% agarose gel electrophoresis (Figure 4.1), and quantity of DNA was estimated on nano drop. The DNA was diluted 200 times in milli Q water (5µl of DNA in 995µl of water) and OD was measured at 260nm and 280nm. One OD at 260 nm of DNA corresponds to 50µg/ml. The concentration of DNA was calculated as DNA (µg/ml) = OD_{260} x Dilution factor x 50. An OD_{260}/OD_{280} ratio in the range of 1.6-2.0 corresponds to an acceptable level of contamination by proteins.

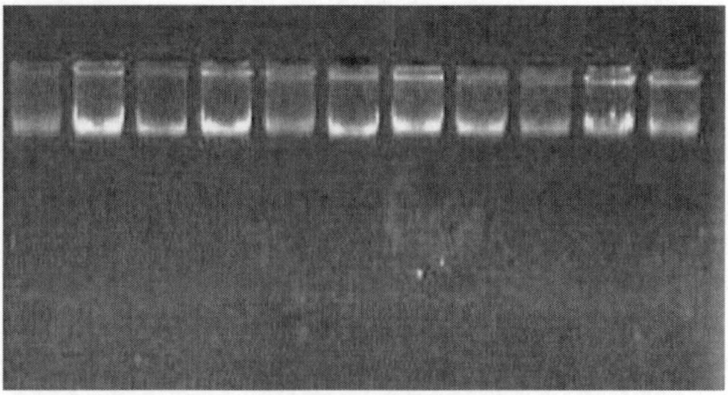

Figure 4.1. 0.8% Agarose gel electrophoresis showing quality of DNA.

4.3.7. Mutation Detection by Polymerase Chain Reaction

The polymerase chain reaction (PCR) technique was used for detecting the polymorphisms of respective genes.

4.3.7.1. Principle

The polymerase chain reaction is a powerful technique in which, the target DNA is amplified in vitro exponentially through an enzymatic reaction of DNA polymerase. The prerequisite for amplification of the desired DNA segment is to know the sequences of template DNA so that the appropriate primer can be tailored. The method employs repeated cycles of denaturation (95^0C), annealing at 50-64^0C of tailored primers to the target DNA, and enzymatic primer extension (72^{0}C) to amplify DNA flanked by the primers. In each subsequent cycle the amplification product serve as templates and hence the process is exponential. Adding the advantages of using thermostable Taq polymerase, it is feasible to perform the amplification process efficiently in an automated system (Figure 4.2.).

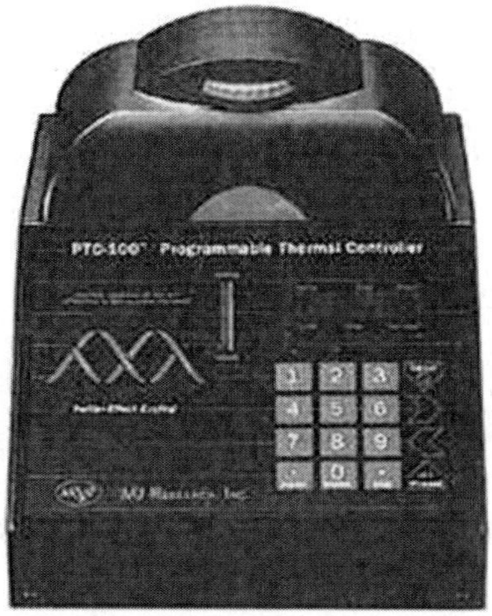

Figure 4.2. Thermal cycler (Bio-Rad PTC 100).

4.3.7.2. PCR Reaction Components

The following components which, performs specific functions are needed to perform the efficient amplification of the target DNA for analysis.

(a) DNA polymerase: The most commonly used enzyme for the DNA polymerization is *Taq* DNA polymerase, which is derived from *Thermus aquaticus* (a bacterium which flourishes in hot springs). This enzyme is heat resistant, with a broad optimal pH of 8.2- 9.0 in 10 mM Tris. One or two units of the enzymes are sufficient to perform a PCR reaction in a final volume of 50μl.

(b) Deoxynucleotide triphosphates (dNTP's): The dNTP's are the second major components of the PCR reaction. These are the building blocks of the newly synthesized DNA (PCR products). However, the dNTP's should not exceed 250μM because excess amount of dNTP's chelates Mg^{++} ions of the PCR mix and gives false incorporation of the nucleotides in the amplification.

(c) Reaction buffer: The reaction buffer provides the environment in which the polymerase works optimally. The buffer components may vary widely according to the DNA template sequence to be amplified. A buffer containing 10mM Tris–HCl (pH 8.4), 1.5mM $MgCl_2$ is generally efficient for amplifying a variety of DNA regions, although $MgCl_2$ concentration often requires optimization.

4.3.7.3. PCR Cycle

There are three major steps in a PCR, which are repeated for 30 or 40 cycles. This is done on an automated Thermo cycler, which can heat or cool the tubes with the reaction mixture in a very short time.

(a) Denaturation (90-94^{0}C): During the denaturation, the double strand melts open to single stranded DNA.

(b) Annealing (50-65^{0}C): During annealing, primers hybridize or "anneal" to their complementary sequences on either side of the target sequence. The primers normally jiggle around due to Brownian motion. Hydrogen bonds are constantly formed and broken between the single stranded primer and the single stranded template. The more stable bonds last a little bit longer and on that little piece of double stranded DNA (template and primer), the polymerase can attach and start copying the template. Once there are few bases built in, the hydrogen bond is so strong between the template and the primer that it does not break anymore.

(c) Extension (72^{0}C): The primers, where there are few bases built in, have a stronger attraction to the template, created by hydrogen bonds, than the forces breaking these attractions. Primers that are on opposite with no exact match get loose again (because of the higher temperature) and don't give extension of the fragment.

4.3.8. Restriction Fragment Length Polymorphism (PCR-RFLP)

Restriction enzymes cut double-stranded DNA at specific recognition sequences. Some mutations naturally create or abolish restriction enzyme sites, in such cases mutant and normal alleles can be distinguished by amplifying across the mutant site and digesting the PCR product with relevant restriction endonucleases and the resulting DNA fragments are separated on gel. The length of the fragment size depends on the presence and absence of the recognition sites in the amplified product. The genotyping for S549N and IVS8-5T was carried out by PCR-RFLP method.

4.3.8.1. SPINK1 Gene Polymorphisms

4.3.8.1a. N34S (101A>G)

N34S polymorphism was studied by PCR-RFLP by Plendl et al. 2001. PCR was performed using Taq DNA polymerase (2.5 U), dNTPs (200 μmol / l each), and 0.4 μmol/l of each primer in a total volume of 50 μl. Cycle conditions were as follows: initial denaturation at 95^{0}C; 35 cycles of 1 min denaturation at 95^{0}C, 1 min of annealing at 65^{0}C and 2 min of primer extension at 72^{0}C; and a final extension for 5 minutes at 72^{0}C. The PCR products were directly digested for at least 2-4 hrs at 65^{0}C with TaaI (MBI, Fermentas) following the recommendation of manufacturers. Digested products were checked on a 2% agarose gel at 80 V, stained with ethidium bromide, and visualized under UV light. For the wild type allele, complete digestion with TaaI produced 4 fragments of 20, 137, 139, and 299 bps. When the mutated allele was present, the 299 bp fragment was cut; resulting into two bands sized 109 and 190 bp. The results are shown in Figure 4.3.

Figure 4.3. 1.5% Agarose gel shows he detection of 101 (A>G) substitution in exon-3 of SPINK 1 gene. Lanes 1, 2, 3 and 4 show wild type homozygous (AA) genotypes. Lanes 6 and 7 show mutant heterozygous (AG) genotype and the mutant homozygous (GG) genotype, respectively. M; molecular weight marker.

4.3.8.1b. IVS3+2T>C

The presence of IVS3+2T and or IVS3+2C alleles was examined by primer-introduced restriction analysis by Kume et al. (2002). The sequence of the primers is 5'CAAATGTTACAATGAACTTAATGGATG-3' (forward) and 5'-GTTTAAAAGAAACTCAAGTTTGTACGC-3' (reverse). The cycle condition was as follows: preheating at 95^0 C for 5 min, followed by 40 cycles of 95^{0}C for 30 sec, 60^{0}C for 30 sec and 72^{0}C for 30 sec; and then a final extension at 72^{0}C for 5 min. The PCR products were digested with HhaI and separated by 3% agarose gel electrophoresis. The unrestricted 134-bp product represents the T allele, whereas the C allele was cut in to 107-bp and 27-bp fragments. The results are shown in Figure 4.4.

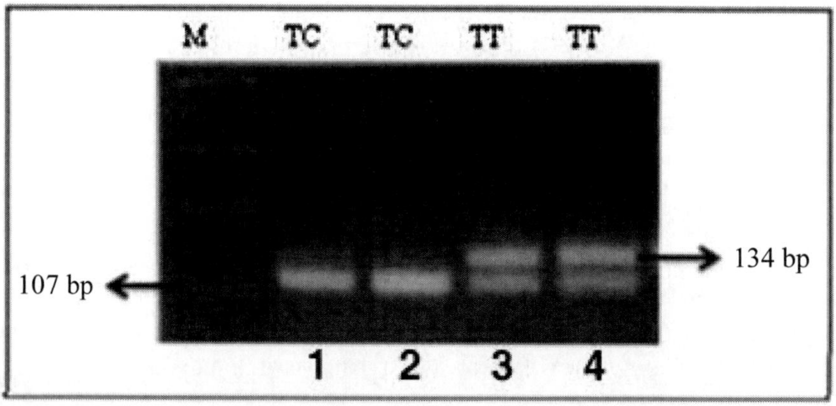

Figure 4.4. 3% Agarose gel showing genotyping of IVSS3+2T>C. Lanes 3 and 4 showing wild type (TT) genotype, Lane 1 and 2 showing mutant heterozygous (TC) genotype and M showing molecular weight marker.

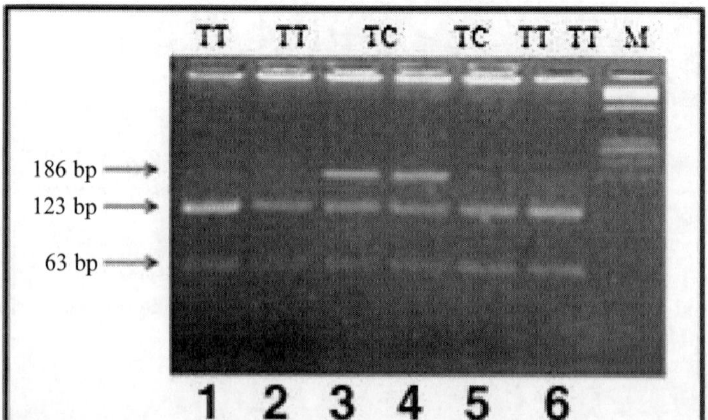

Figure 4.5. 3% Agarose gel shows detection of IVS1 (37T>C) substitution in intron 1 of SPINK1 gene. Lanes 1, 2, 5 and 6 show wild type homozygous (TT) genotype, Lanes 3 and 4 show mutant heterozygous (TC) genotype. The mutant homozygous (CC) genotype was not detected in either the patient or control. M; molecular weight marker.

4.3.8.1c. IVS1-37T>C

The presence of IVS1-37T and or IVS1-37C alleles was examined by primer-introduced restriction analysis by Yuji Ota et al. (2010). The cycle conditions were as follows: preheating at 95°C for 2 min; followed by 20 (for the initial amplification) cycles of 95°C for 30 s, 60°C for 30 s, and 72°C for 30 s, and then a final extension at 72°C for 5 min. The amplified PCR product (186 bp) was subjected for digestion with Dde1 restriction enzyme. The fragments of 123 bp and 63 bp represent the wild type allele. However, abolition of restriction enzyme sites indicates the presence of mutant allele. The results are shown in Figure 4.5.

4.3.9. Amplification Refractory Mutation System (ARMS-PCR)

Newton et al described the amplification refractory mutation system (ARMS) as a general technique for the analysis of any point mutation or small deletion. It is a simple, rapid, non isotopic and reliable method, and results can be obtained in a single working day. The principle behind this method is that oligonucleotides which are complementary to a given DNA sequence except for a mismatch at their 3'-OH residue will not function as primers in the PCR under appropriate conditions [Newton et al. 1989].

A typical ARMS test consists of two complementary reactions.

1. Normal reaction: Contains primer specific for the normal DNA sequence and cannot amplify mutant DNA at a given locus.
2. Mutant reaction: Contains a mutant-specific primer for the mutant DNA sequence and does not amplify normal DNA at a given locus.

The genotype of an individual is determined by analysis of the length of the amplification products.

1. Wild-type homozygote: Generates PCR product only with the primers having normal sequences.
2. Heterozygote: Generates PCR product with normal and mutant primers both.
3. Mutant- type homozygote: Generates PCR product only with mutant primers.

4.3.9.1. CFTR Gene Mutation

All cases and controls were screened for five common *CFTR* gene variants identified worldwide (ΔF508, G542X, G551D, R117H) Peripheral blood (3.0 ml) was collected in EDTA vial and DNA extraction was done using standard Phenol-chloroform method. Mutation Analysis was done using ARMS-PCR, described by *Ferrie et al. (1992)* and PCR-RFLP method was used for S549N and IVS8-5T polymorphism. For quality control samples of subjects identified as mutant and 10% of the randomly selected samples were genotyped once again to rule out any inconsistency. The list of primers and PCR conditions used are shown in Table 4.1.

Table 4.1. Primers and PCR conditions used for detection of ΔF508, G551D, G542X, R117H mutations

S No	Mutation/ Location/ Predicted effect	Primers Sequence (5' - 3')		PCR condition (Annealing temp°C/ Extension time in sec/ number of cycles)	PCR product size (bp)
1	ΔF508/ Exon 10/ Deletion Phe-508	C	GACTTCACTTCTAATGATGATTATGGGAG	60/ 120/ 35	N-160 M-157
		N	GTATCTATATTCATCATAGGAAACACCAC		
		M	GTATCTATATTCATCATAGGAAACACCAT		
2	G551D/ Exon 11/ Gly-551→Asp	C	TAAAATTTCAGCAATGTTGTTTTTGACC	60/ 120/ 35	N-285 M-286
		N	GCTAAAGAAATTCTTGCTCGTTGCC		
		M	AGCTAAAGAAATTCTTGCTCGTTGCT		
3	G542X/ Exon 11/ Gly-542→Stop	C	TAAAATTTCAGCAATGTTGTTTTTGACC	60/ 120/ 35	N-256 M-257
		N	ACTCAGTGTGATTCCACCTTCTAC		
		M	CACTCAGTGTGATTCCACCTTCTCA		
4	R117H/ Exon4/ Arg-117-His	C	CACATATGGTATGACCCTCTATATAAACT	60/120/35	N-237 M-237
		N	CCTATGCCTAGATAAATCGCGATAGAAC		
		M	CCTATGCCTAGATAAATCGCGATAGAAT		
		N	CCTGTGGTATCACTCCAAAGGCTTTCCAC		
		M	CCTGTGGTATCACTCCAAAGGCTTTCCAT		

* Arg, Arginine; Asp, Asparagine; Gly, Glycine; His, Histidine; Phe, Phenylalanine; Trp, Tryptophan.

4.3.9.1a. ΔF508

It is the most common mutation in the CFTR gene. There is three-base-pair deletion (CTT) that produces an in-frame deletion of a phenylalanine (F) at position 508 (NBD1 domain). It belongs to Class II mutations of CFTR gene. It gives amplification of 160bp in normal reaction and 157bp in mutant reaction. The results are shown in Figure 4.6.

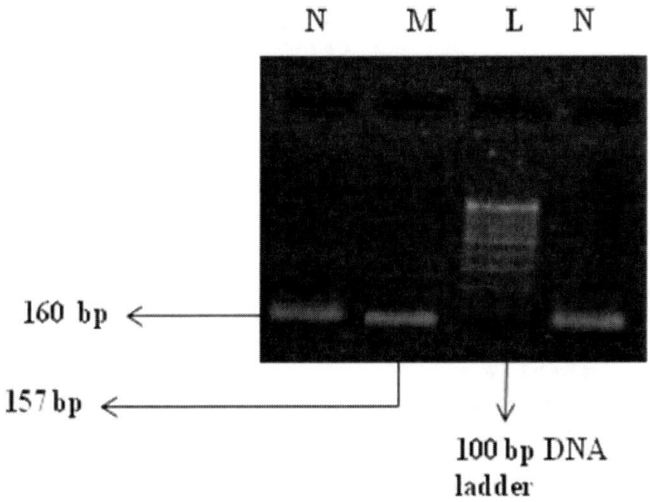

Figure 4.6. Gel picture representing ΔF508 mutation (normal-160bp, mutant-157 bp) of CFTR gene, where N; Normal, M; Mutant, L; 100 base pair DNA ladder, bp; base pair.

4.3.9.1b. G542X

It is a nonsense mutation (class I), G→T transition at nucleotide 1756 in exon 11, results in the mutation of codon (GGA) for the amino acid glycine at 542 to the translational stop codon TGA. It belongs to Class I mutations of CFTR gene. It gives amplification of 256bp in normal reaction and 257bp in mutant reaction. The results are shown in Figure 4.7.

4.3.9.1c. G5551D

It is a missense mutation in which a G→A transition at nucleotide1784 in exon11, results in Glycine to Aspartic acid substitution at amino acid 551. It belongs to Class III mutations of CFTR gene. It gives amplification of 285bp in normal reaction and 286bp in mutant reaction. The results are shown in Figure 4.8.

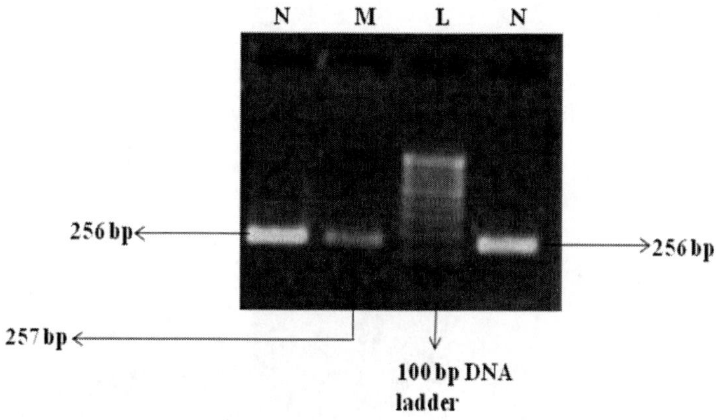

Figure 4.7. Gel picture representing G542X mutation (normal-256 bp, mutant-257 bp) of CFTR gene where N; Normal, M; Mutant, L; 100 base pair DNA ladder, bp; base pair.

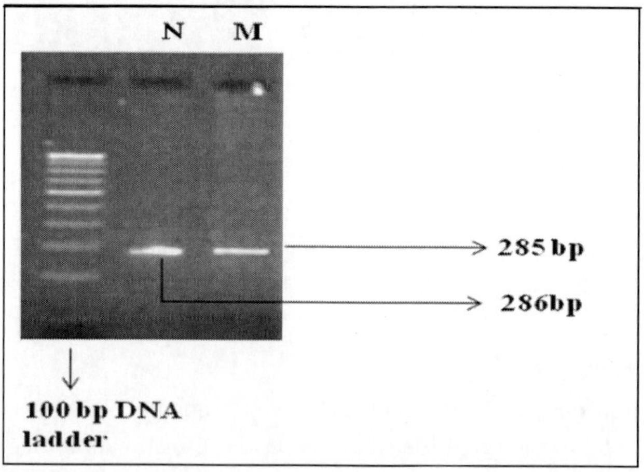

Figure 4.8. Gel picture representing G551D mutation (normal-285 bp, mutant-286 bp) of CFTR gene, where N; Normal, M; Mutant, L; 100 base pair DNA ladder, bp; base pair.

4.3.9.1d. R117H

It is a missense mutation in which a G→A transition at nucleotide 984 in exon4, results in Arginine to Histidine substitution at amino acid 117. It belongs to Class IV mutations of CFTR gene. It gives amplification of 237bp in normal reaction and 237bp in mutant reaction. The results are shown in Figure 4.9.

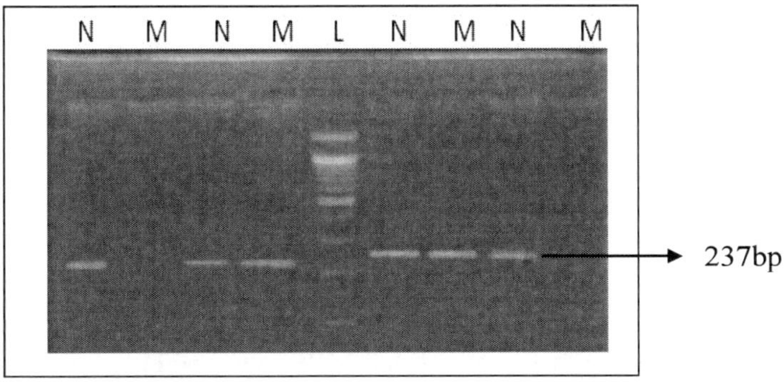

Figure 4.9. Gel picture representing R117H mutation (normal-237 bp, mutant-237 bp) of CFTR gene, where N; Normal, M; Mutant, L; 100 base pair DNA ladder, bp; base pair.

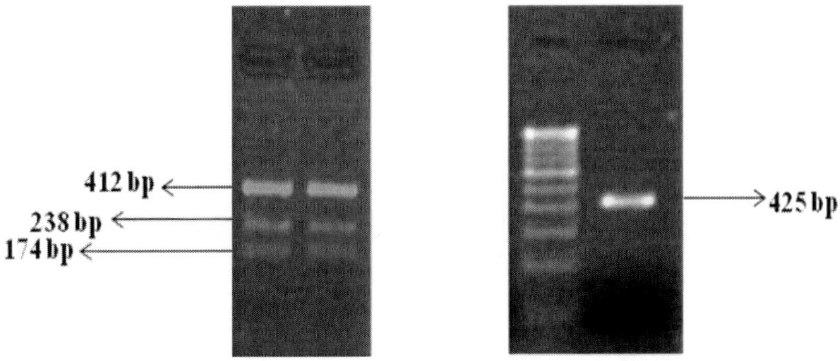

Figure 4.10. Gel picture representing the S549N mutation of the CFTR gene.

4.3.9.1e. S549N

Exon 11 was amplified using the primers, forward: CAA CTG TGG TTA AAG CAA TAG TGT and reverse: GCA CAG ATT CTG AGT AAC CAT AAT [Apostol et al. 2009]. PCR condition was as follows: Initial denaturation at 94°C for 6 min and then 30 cycles of denaturation (94°C for 30 sec), primer annealing (55°C for 30 sec), and extension (72°C for 60 sec) followed by a final extension period of 7 min. The reaction mixture contained 2.5 μl of 10X buffer; 200 *m*M of each dNTPs (dATP, dCTP, dTTP and dGTP); 20 pmol of each primer; and 1 unit of *Taq* DNA polymerase in a final volume of 25 µl, containing 100 ng of genomic DNA. The final PCR products (425 bp) were digested with Dde I enzyme and visualized on 3% agarose gel. The digested normal PCR product yielded the fragment of 238 bp, 174 bp, 13 bp and mutant produced fragments of 412 bp and 13 bp. The results are shown in Figure 4.10.

4.3.9.1f. 5T Allele of Intron 8

Exon 9 was first amplified with primers, forward: TAA TGG ATC ATG GGC CAT GT and reverse: ACA GTG TTG AAT GTG GTG CA [Chillon et al. 1995]. The PCR conditions were as follows: denaturation at 95°C for 30 seconds, annealing at 54°C for 30 seconds, and extension at 74°C for 40 seconds, for 25 cycles. The reaction mixture contained 2.5μl of 10X buffer; 200 mM of each dNTPs (dATP, dCTP, dTTP and dGTP); 20 pmol of each primer; and 1 unit of *Taq* DNA polymerase in a final volume of 25μl, containing 100 ng of genomic DNA. To amplify the polypyrimidine sequence while avoiding the adjacent dinucleotide repeat (TG)n, nested PCR was performed with primers, forward: CCGCCGCTGTGTGTGTGTGTGTGTTT TT and reverse: GGATCCAGCAACCGCCAACA. The conditions of the nested PCR were similar as described above except that 1μl of amplified product of first PCR reaction served as template. The nested PCR was performed for 35 cycles. The final PCR products (203 bp) were digested with Xmn I enzyme and visualized on 12 percent non-denaturing polyacrylamide gel/ 4% agarose gel after electrophoresis for four to five hours at 180 V. In case of 5T allele digested PCR product yields fragments of 84 bp and 119 bp. The poly T tract consists of three alleles 5T, 7T and 9T. Where the most common genotype combination in the population is 7T homozygosity followed by 9T. Since our concern was to assess association of 5T allele with chronic pancreatitis, the individuals with the genotype combination 5T/5T, 5T/7T and 5T/9T have been considered as mutant and individuals with the genotype combination 7T/7T, 9T/9T and 7T/9T as wild type for statistical analysis. The results are shown in Figure 4.11.

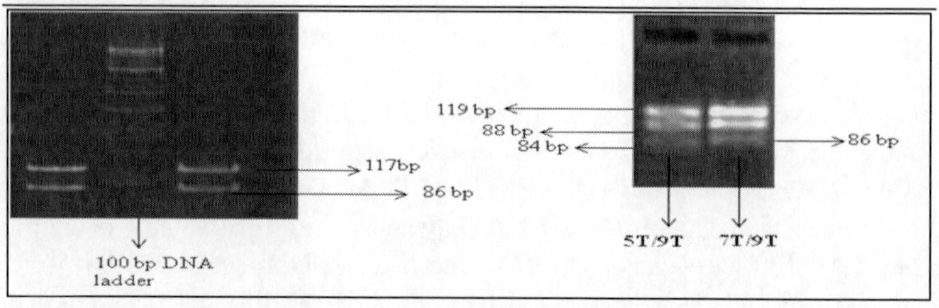

Figure 4.11. Gel picture representing poly T alleles in the intron 8 of CFTR gene.

4.3.9.2. Cathepsin B Gene Polymorphism

The restriction enzyme (Rsa I) digestion of Leu26Val (C76G) PCR products and their separation is shown in Figure 6.9 by *Mahurkar et al. 2006*. The digestion of PCR product (238bp) produces 215bp and 23bp fragments for wild type alleles whereas, undigested product indicates presence of mutant allele. The amplification protocol consisted of an initial denaturation segment at 94^{0}C for 5 min, after this each cycle consisted of three segments denaturation at 94^{0}C for 30 sec, annealing at 65^{0}C for 40 sec, extension at 72^{0}C for 45 sec). The cycle was repeated 35 times followed by an additional final extension at 72^{0}C for 10 min. The PCR products were resolved on 2.0% of agarose gel. The results are shown in Figure 4.12.

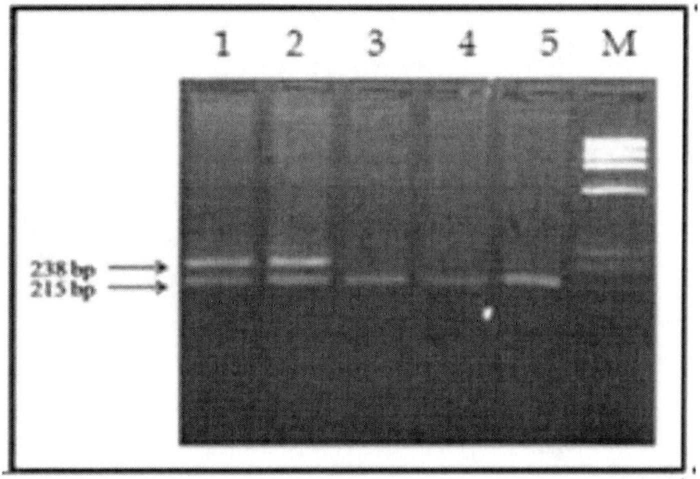

Figure 4.12. 3% Agarose gel shows detection of Leu26Val (CG) mutation in exon 3 of Cathepsin B gene. Lanes 1 and 2 show heterozygous (CG) genotype. Lanes 3, 4 and 5 show wild type (CC) genotype. The mutant homozygous (GG) genotype was not detected. M; molecular weight marker.

4.3.9.3. Methylene Tetrahydrofolate Reductase (MTHFR) C677T Polymorphism

The identification of C to T transition at nucleotide 677 was done using the methods Frost et al. (1995). The amplification protocol consisted of an initial denaturation segment at 94^{0}C for 4 min after this each cycle consisted of three segments (denaturation at 94^{0}C for 30 sec, annealing at 62^{0}C for 45 sec, extension at 72^{0}C for 45 sec). The cycle was repeated 30 times followed by an additional final extension at 72^{0}C for 12 min. The PCR products were checked on 2.0% of agarose gel. A band of 198 bp was observed under transilluminator by staining with 1μg/ml of ethidium bromide. 10μL of the PCR products were aliquoted in separate tubes for RFLP to which 10 units of the restriction enzyme HinfI was added and kept at 37^{0}C for 6-8 hours. The digested products were checked in 3% of agarose gel and visualized under transilluminator by ethidium bromide staining. In the case of wild type allele undigested band of 198 bp was observed. While in the condition of mutant allele a band of 175bp was observed as the presence of restriction site. The results are shown in Figure 4.13.

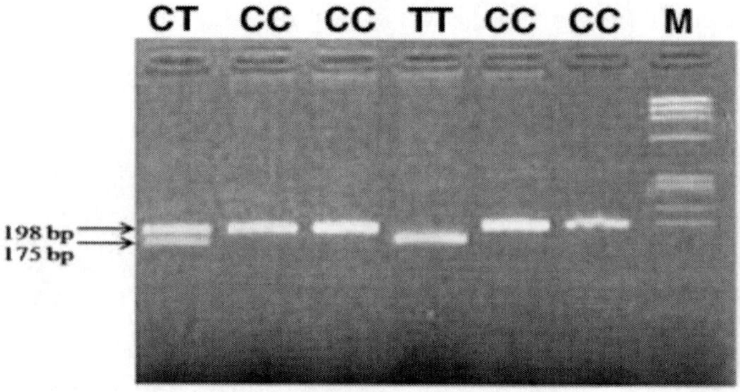

Figure 4.13. 3% Agarose gel showing Genotyping of MTHFR. Lanes 2, 3, 5 and 6 show wild type (CC) genotype, lane 1 show mutant heterozygous (CT) genotype and lane 4 show mutant homozygous (TT) genotype, M showing molecular weight Marker.

4.3.9.4. Angiotensin Converting ENZYME (ACE) I/D Gene Polymorphism

The ACE I/D polymorphism was genotyped using polymerase chain reaction (PCR) by Berge et al. (1997). The amplification protocols were initial denaturation at 95^{0}C for 5 min followed by 30 cycles each of denaturation at 97^{0}C for 45 sec, annealing of primers at 60^{0}C for 1 min 15 sec and extension at 72^{0}C for 2 min 30 sec and final extension at 72^{0}C for 5 min. The PCR products were 490 bp for allele insertion (I) and 198 bp for deletion (D) allele. PCR products were separated on 1.5% of agarose gel and visualized under transilluminator by staining with 1μg/ml of ethidium bromide. The results are shown in Figure 4.14.

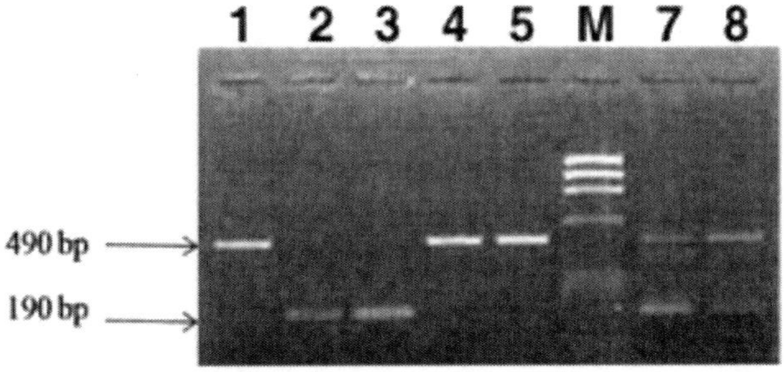

Figure 4.14. Amplified products for ACE polymorphism. Lanes 1, 4 and 5 show II genotype, lanes 2 and 3 show DD genotype, lanes 7 and 8 show ID genotype, M shows molecular marker.

4.4. Methodology for Family Screening

Family screening was done for 10 families' subjects'. Addresses and contact numbers were taken at the time of recruitment. Telephone calls were done and letters were sent to the families, whose proper addresses and numbers were available. 2 ml venous blood sample was collected in EDTA vial from each member and DNA was extracted using standard phenol-chloroform method. Genotyping was done by methods following the conditions of PCR-RFLP and ARMS method.

4.5. Data Entry and Statistical Analysis

4.5.1. Data Entry

Date was entered in Micro Soft Excel. It was double entered and manually cleaned.

4.5.2. Data Analysis

Data was analyzed using software Statistical software for Social Sciences (SPSS, Version 17, Chicago, Illinois, USA) and EPI6. Chi- square and Students t-test were used to test the association between categorical and continuous variables. Fisher's exact test was used if expected cell frequencies were lower than 5. Statistical inferences were based on the conventional level of statistical significance ($P < 0.05$).

4.5.3. Genotype Frequency

Genotype frequency is the frequency or proportion of a genotype on a genetic locus in a population. It was calculated as number of individuals with a given genotype divided by the total number of individuals in population and expressed as a percentage.

4.5.4. Allele Frequency

Allele frequency is the measure of relative frequency of an allele on a genetic locus in a population. It was calculated as the number of copies of a particular allele divided by the number of copies of all alleles at the genetic locus.

4.5.5. Odds Ratio (OR)

Risk or protection for disease due to presence of particular genotype or allele was calculated using Odds ratio. The odds ratio is ratio of odds of exposure in diseased subjects to the odds of exposure in the non-diseased. For each variant the contingency table (2x2) was constructed as shown below:

	Cases	Controls	Total
Mutation present	A	B	A+B
Mutation absent	C	D	C +D
Total	A+ C	B+ D	A+B+ C+D

The odds in the cases and controls were calculated as shown below:

$$\text{Odds Ratio} = {}^{(A/B)}/_{(C/D)} = (A \times D) / (B \times C)$$

The odds ratio takes values between zero ('0') and infinity. One ('1') is the neutral value and means that there is no difference between the groups compared; close to zero or infinity means a large difference. An odds ratio greater than 1 means cases carrying mutation have more risk for the disease and less than 1 means cases carrying mutation are protective for the disease.

4.5.6. Hardy–Weinberg Equilibrium (HWE)

G.H. Hardy (the English Mathematician) and W. Weinberg (the German Physician) independently worked out the mathematical basis of population genetics in 1908. It describes and predicts genotype and allele frequencies in a non-evolving population. The Hardy-Weinberg principle states that in a large randomly breeding population, both genotype and allele frequencies will remain constant from generation to generation assuming that there is no mutation, gene migration, selection or genetic drift. Their formula predicts the expected genotype frequencies using the allele frequencies in a diploid Mendelian population.

$$p^2+2pq+q^2=1$$

It describes the binomial distribution of genotypes that result in a population when there are no external pressures that cause deviation from $p^2+2pq+q^2$. In this formula, p^2 corresponds to the frequency of homozygous genotype AA, 2pq to Aa and q^2 to aa. The AA, Aa, aa were the three possible genotypes for a biallelic locus. If the difference between observed and expected frequency was >0.05 using chi-square goodness of test statistics, the population for that genotype was considered in HWE.

Alleles that are causative of disease would be expected to be disproportionately over-represented among cases than controls. Deviation from HWE might provide clue to the role of genes in etiology of the disease.

HWE in control population was assessed online (http://www.genes.org.uk/software/hardy-weinberg.html) and *p*-value was considered significant at <0.05 level.

Chapter 5

RESULTS OBTAINED FROM THE STUDY ON MOLECULAR ANALYSES OF TROPICAL CHRONIC PANCREATITIS

The present study included 150 cases of TCP and 150 age and sex matched controls from October 2009 to March 2013. Figure 5.1 represents the number of patients recruited each month over a period of 3 years. The maximum numbers of patient were recorded in the months of April and May. Mean age of patients was 49.9 ± 14.8 year, falling in the range of 10-55 years. Of which 56.6% were male and 43.4% were female.

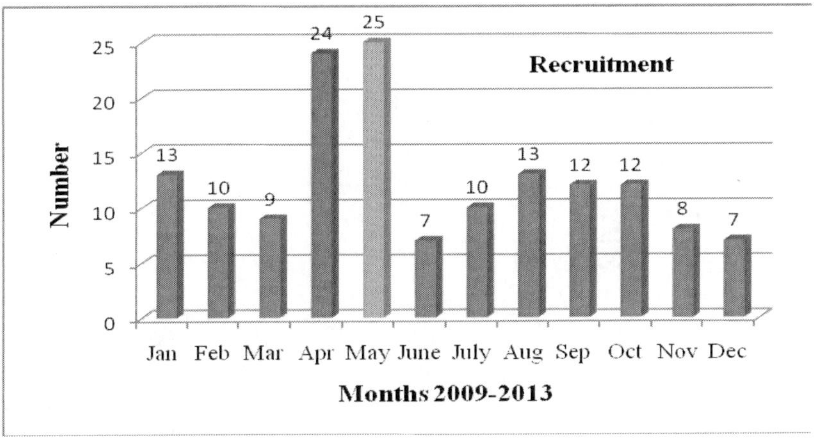

Figure 5.1. Average number of patients recruited each month.

Figure 5.2 represents the categorization of patients on the basis of age at recruitment in years, with maximum number of patients in the age group of 20 to 40 years. The age of presentation shows the occurrence of disease in second decade.

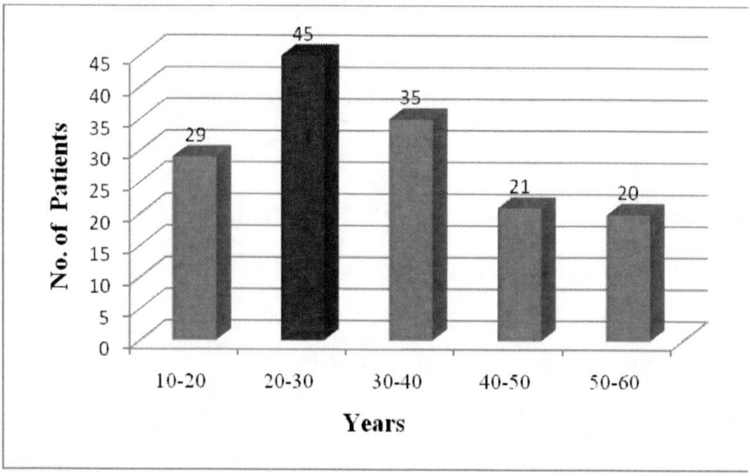

Figure 5.2. Categorization of patients on the basis of age recruitment in years.

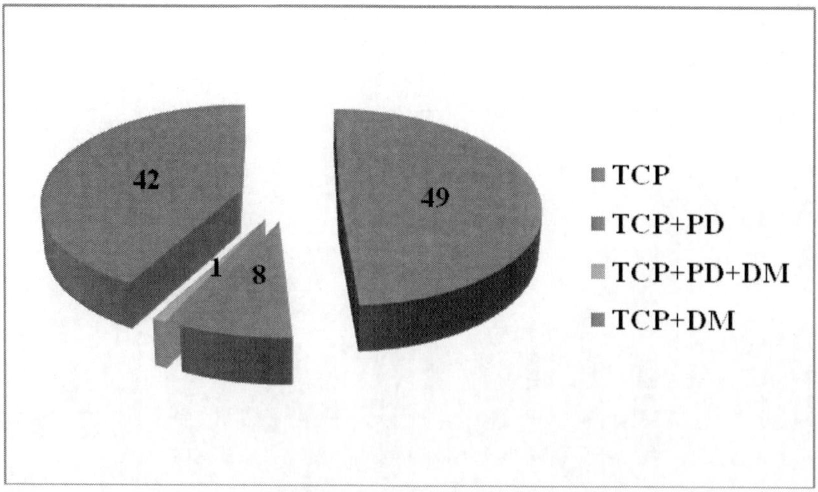

Figure 5.3 Number of subjects studied in cases with category distribution.

5.1. Category Distribution of TCP Patients

The 150 cases of TCP patients were further categorized in various groups like: 49% of TCP patients with no other clinical complications, 42% of TCP with Diabetes Mellitus with exocrine / endocrine insufficiency, 8% TCP with Pancreas Divisum (PD) and 1% of CP with pancreas divisum plus diabetes mellitus. Though PD itself is not a cause of pancreatitis but it is one of the important clinical finding of TCP. These four groups are shown in Figure 5.3.

5.1.1. Region Wise Distribution of Tropical Chronic Pancreatitis Patients

The geographical distribution of TCP patients was also a reflection of the etiologies of the disease. 8% of the patients were from Basti and 7% from Gorakhpur. The results presented in Figure 5.4 showed that there was common denominator of the region, which reflects the poor standard of nutrition. Moreover, the climate of this region is favourable in progression of disease. Large segments of population in this region use insufficient amount of protein in their diet. Further, the quality of their lives is relatively poor. So the factors closely associated with quality, environment, diet and congenital abnormality increase the threat of the disease. As the number of patients recruited was less, so it does not reflect the overall frequency.

5.1.2. Categorization of Patients (a) and Controls (b) into Three Groups

The TCP patients (150) and controls (150) were further classified into three groups; depicted in Figures 5.5 and 5.6. Group I consisted of diabetics/non diabetics, group II contained smokers/Nonsmokers and group III consisted of family history/no family history of TCP. The ratio of diabetics/non-diabetics was 42:49 in TCP as compared to 28:72 in control groups. The percentage of smokers in TCP group was 39.3% more than the control group.

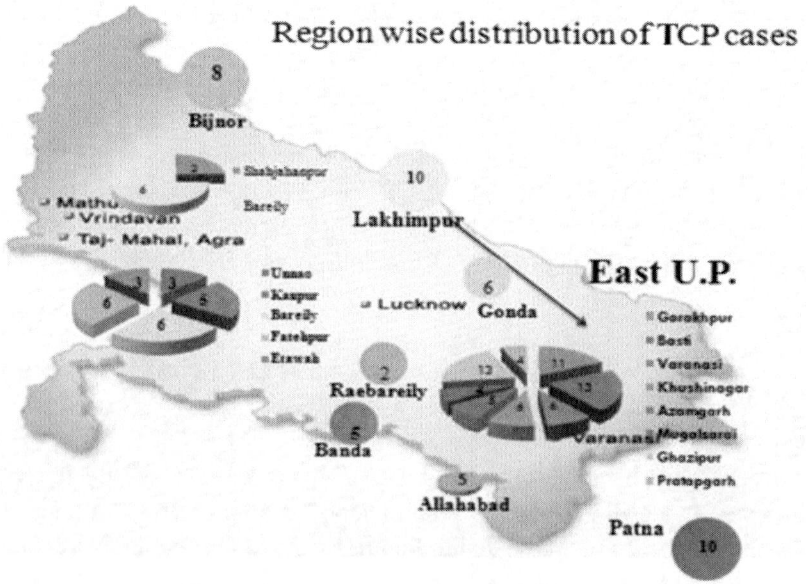

Figure 5.4. Regional distribution of recruited TCP patients.

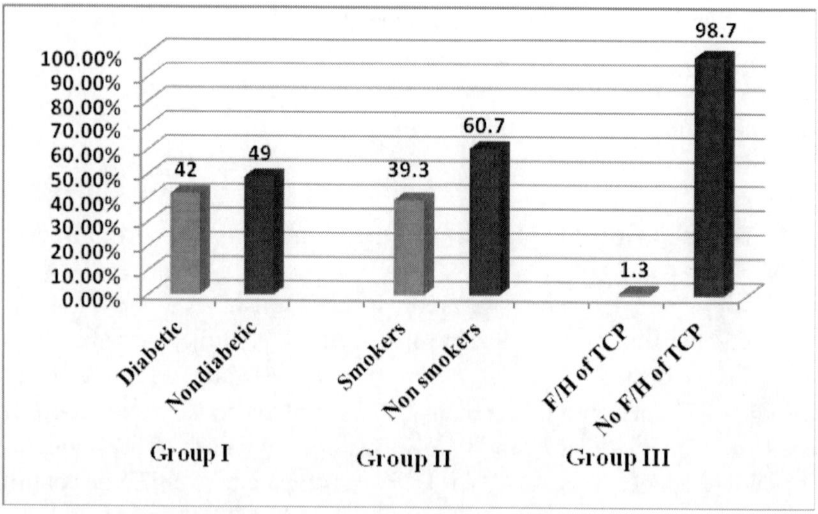

Figure 5.5. TCP Patient group.

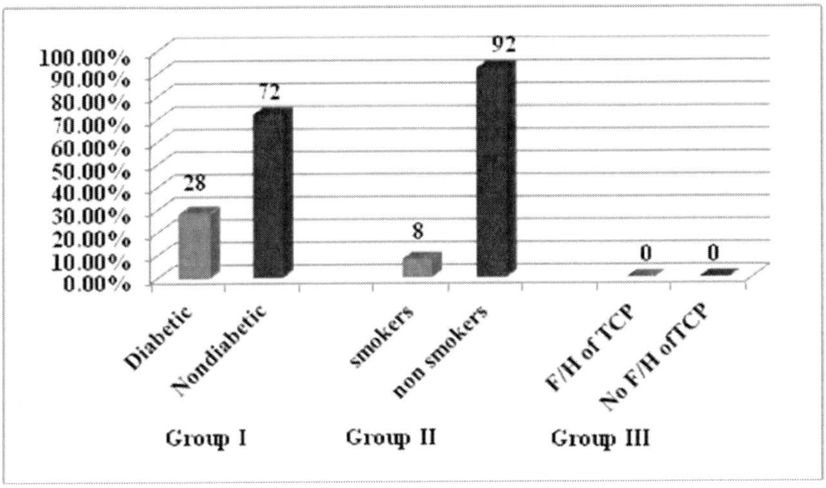

Figure 5.6. Control group.

The number of individuals having classical risk factors viz diabetes; smoking and family history were found to be significantly higher in patients group shown in Figure 5.7.

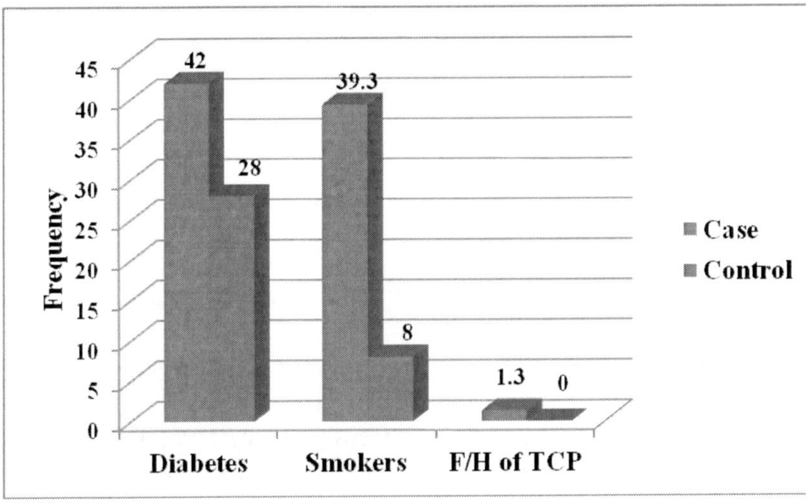

Figure 5.7. Comparison of TCP and control group.

5.1.3. Demographic and Biochemical Profiles of Controls and Patients

The present study includes 105 males and 45 females in the TCP group, and 104 healthy males and 46 healthy females in control group. This shows an insignificant difference in male: female ratio in both the groups. However, a significant (p=0.001) difference for mean values of BMI and weight were noted between TCP patients and controls (Table 5.1).

Table 5.1. Demographic and biochemical profile of controls and patients

Characteristics	Controls	TCP cases	P- value
N	150	150	-
Age	36.86±1.23	34.86±1.183	0.217
Sex (M:F)	104:46	105:45	0.892
Weight (kg)	68.19±9.634	56.23±13.230	0.001
BMI (wt/ht2)	25.16±3.15	23.3±3.25	0.001
Diabetic:nondiabetic	42:108	59:91	0.030
Smoker: nonsmoker	12:138	55:95	0.000
Alcohalic:non-alcoholic	9:141	13:137	0.333
Triglyceride (45-150 mg/dL)	154.62±39.37	170.34±49.61	0.131
Total Cholesterol (125-250mg/dL)	95.34±27.47	151.18±43.03	0.001
HDL-cholesterol (23-60mg/dL)	39.34 ±7.79	36.62±7.678	0.023
LDL-cholesterol (92-148mg/dL)	38.41±7.76	86.35±31.11	0.002
VLDL- cholesterol (10-30mg/dL)	19.54±6.61	25.96±12.22	0.023

Mean±SD, Unpaired t-test, N=Number.

A complete lipid profile like: triglycerides, total cholesterol, HDL cholesterol, LDL cholesterol and VLDL cholesterol in controls and patients are shown in Table 5.1. The values of total cholesterol, triglyceride (TG), very low density lipoprotein (VLDL) and low density lipoprotein (LDL) were found significantly higher in CP patients than in controls with significant association. However, the level of High density lipoprotein (HDL) was found lower in TCP patients group. A higher % of smokers and diabetes were observed in patients group (p<0.001) compared to controls.

Table 5.2. The age of onset of disease, age of presentation and duration of the symptom

TCP patients (n)	150
Males (%)	70
Females (%)	30
Age (years; means ±s.d.)	49.9±14.8
Age at diagnosis(years; mean±s.d)	35.8±16.7
Age of onset (years; means±s.d)	26.04±9.82
Age of onset of pain (years; means±s.d)	30.8±14.56
Age (mean) at presentation calcific /non-calcific	30.5/23 =1.3
Pain (%)	65.3
Duration of pain calcific /non-calcific (Years)	2.19
Smokers (%)	39
No. of cigarettes (cig/day; mean±s.d)	19.1±13.4
BMI (kg/m2; mean±s.d.)	23.3±3.25
Age of onset of DM (means±s.d)	36.2±11.27
Complications of diabetes calcific /non-calcific (%)	1.22
Colelithiasis (%)	16.5
Dyslipidemia (%)	5.2
Pancreas divisum (%)	8
Autoimmune TCP (%)	1.5
Obstructive TCP (%)	9.3
Calcification (%)	53.5
Pseudo cysts (%)	29.6
Steatorrhea (%)	4.3

5.1.4. Clinical Features of Patient Group

The male to female ratio in TCP patients was 2.3:1.0. The mean age of diagnosis was found 35.8±16.7. The presentation of the disease was 30.5 years in the calcific group and 23 years in the non-calcific group. Pain was the commonest presenting symptom, and it was present in 65% of patients. The age of onset of diabetes mellitus was 36.2±11.27 years. The duration of pain in calcific and non calcific groups was found 2.19 years. The age of onset of disease and the presentation and duration of the symptom are given in Table 5.2. In addition, calcification was observed in 54% of patients. Steatorrhea was observed in 4.3%. Coleolithiasis was observed in 16.5% of cases. The history of all the patients indicate the age of onset of the disease 26.04±9.8, which is quiet early but confound diagnosis was usually established at later stages of life i.e.35.8±16.7 years. Cigarettes smoking was found quiet common in 39% of cases and diabetes get precipitated in second and third decade of life in CP patients, that leads to complications in duration of calcification and pain (Table 5.2).

The diabetes related complications in TCP patients are given in Table 5.3. The presence of ketosis, neuropathy and tuberculosis. Neuropathy and tuberculosis were present in 1% and 2% of patients.

Table 5.3. Diabetes-complications

Complications	Percentage
Ketosis	2
Hypoglycemic episodes	-
K.W. Syndrome	-
Neuropathy	1
Retinopathy	-
Tuberculosis	2

In our studied subjects none of TCP patients died in their thirties as a result of neuropathy or infections. Nearly 10% of TCP patients had to undergo surgery mostly for intractable pain occurring due to formation of pseudo cysts or common bile duct obstruction. Only 42% of TCP patients developed diabetes mellitus type2 during the course of study.

5.2. Molecular Analysis

Molecular analysis of TCP patients were carried out in order to assess the type and frequency of SPINK1, CFTR, Cathepsin B, ACE and MTHFR gene polymorphism in both the groups i.e. chronic pancreatitis and controls.

5.2.1. Genotype and Allele Frequency of SPINK1 Gene

The genotype and allele frequency of SPINK 1 gene was carried out in 150 cases of TCP and 150 cases of controls. All the samples were tested for three polymorphism N34S, IVS3+2T>C and IVS1-37T>C by PCR-RRFLP method described by Plendal et al.2001, Kume et al. 2002 and Yuji Ota et al. 2010, respectively.

5.2.1.1. 101A>G Polymorphism

Among 150 cases, 55.3 % (83) were of wild type genotype, 41.3(62) were of heterozygous and 3.3 % (05) were of homozygous. Similarly in 150 controls, 98 % (147) were of wild type genotype, 2% (3) were of heterozygous and no homozygous mutation were found. Heterozygous AG mutation was found to be associated with thirty six times increased risk of CP in comparison to Control (p=0.001; OR=36.60). The results are shown in Figure 5.8. A significant difference was observed between two groups OR: 36.60, 95%CI: 11.13-120.29, p-value: 0.001. The G allele frequency was found 24% (72) in cases as compared to 1% (3) in controls. The results are shown in Figure 5.9. A significant association was observed in the frequency distribution of mutant allele with 19.4 times risk of disease with OR: 19.43, 95% CI 1.06-356.05, p-value 0.006. The results are shown in Table 5.4.

5.2.1.2. IVS3+2T>C Polymorphism

The analysis was performed in 150 cases of which 93.3% (140) were of wild type genotype, 6.7 (10) were of heterozygous and no homozygous mutation was found. Similarly in 150 controls, 99.3 % (149) were of wild type genotype, 0.67 % (1) were of heterozygous and no homozygous mutation were found. The results are shown in Figure 5.10. The heterozygous TC genotype was found to be significantly associated with increased risk of CP ten times as compared to control with odds ratio of 10.6. A significant association was observed in the frequency distribution of heterozygous genotype with OR: 10.6, 95%CI: 1.34-84.26, p-value: 0.014. The frequency of mutant allele C was found 3.3% (10) in cases as compared to 0.3 % (1) in controls. The results are shown in Figure 5.11. Significant association with mutant allele to TCP was observed as compared to controls with OR: 10.3, 95% CI 1.31-81.0, p-value 0.014. The results are shown in Table 5.4.

5.2.1.3. IVS1-37T>C Polymorphism

The analysis was performed on 150 cases in which 92.7% (139) were of wild type genotype, 7.3(11) were of heterozygous and no homozygous was found. Similarly in 150 controls, 99.3 % (149) were of wild type genotype, 0.67 % (1) were of heterozygous and no homozygous were found. The results are shown in Figure 5.12. The heterozygous TC genotype was found to be associated with increased risk of TCP. A significant association was observed in the frequency distribution of heterozygous genotype with OR: 11.38, 95%CI: 1.45-88.75, p-value: 0.008. The frequency of mutant allele C was found 3.7% (11) in cases as compared to 0.3 % (1) in controls. The mutant increase 3.7 times risk of CP. The results are shown in Figure 5.13. A significant association was observed with mutant allele to CP as compared to controls OR: 11.3, 95% CI 1.45-88.7, p-value 0.008. The results are shown in Table 5.4.

Table 5.4. Genotype and allele Frequency of SPINK1 gene Polymorphisms

Polymorphisms	**Type**	**TCP (n=150) (%)**	**Cont (n=150) (%)**	**OR (95% CI) p-value**
101A>G Genotypes	Wild (AA)	83 (55.3)	147 (98)	Reference
	Heterozygous(AG)	62 (41.3)	03 (2)	36.60(11.13-120.29)0.001*
	Mutant (GG)	05 (3.3)	0	19.43(1.06-356.05)0.006*
101A>G Alleles	Wild allele (A)	228 (76)	297 (99)	Reference
	Mutant allele (G)	72 (24)	3 (1)	31.26 (9.72-100.53) 0.001*
IVS3+2T>C Genotypes	Wild (TT)	140 (93.3)	149 (99.3)	Reference
	Heterozygous (TC)	10 (6.7)	1 (0.67)	10.6(1.34-84.26)0.014*
IVS3+2T>C Alleles	Wild allele (T)	290 (96.7)	299 (99.7)	Reference
	Mutant allele (C)	10 (3.3)	1 (0.3)	10.3 (1.31-81.0) 0.014*
IVS1-37T>C Genotypes	Wild (TT)	139 (92.7)	149 (99.3)	Reference
	Heterozygous (TC)	11(7.3)	1 (0.67)	11.38(1.45-88.75)0.008*
IVS1-37T>C Alleles	Wild allele (T)	289 (96.3)	299 (99.7)	Reference
	Mutant allele (C)	11 (3.7)	1 (0.3)	11.38 (1.45-88.7) 0.008*

5.3. Genotype and Allele Frequency of CFTR Gene

The genotype and allele frequency of CFTR gene was carried out in 150 cases of TCP and 150 cases of controls. All the samples were tested for four mutations and two polymorphisms ΔF508, G542X, G551D, R117H, S549N and 5Tby ARMS PCR and PCR-RFLP method described by Ferrie et al. 1992, Chillon et al. 1995 and Apostol et al. 2009.

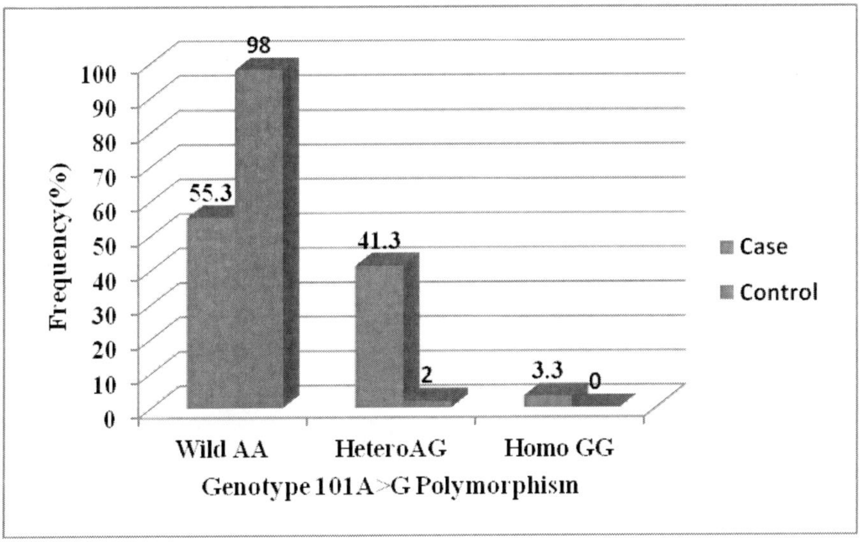

Figure 5.8. Genotype frequency of 101A>G polymorphism.

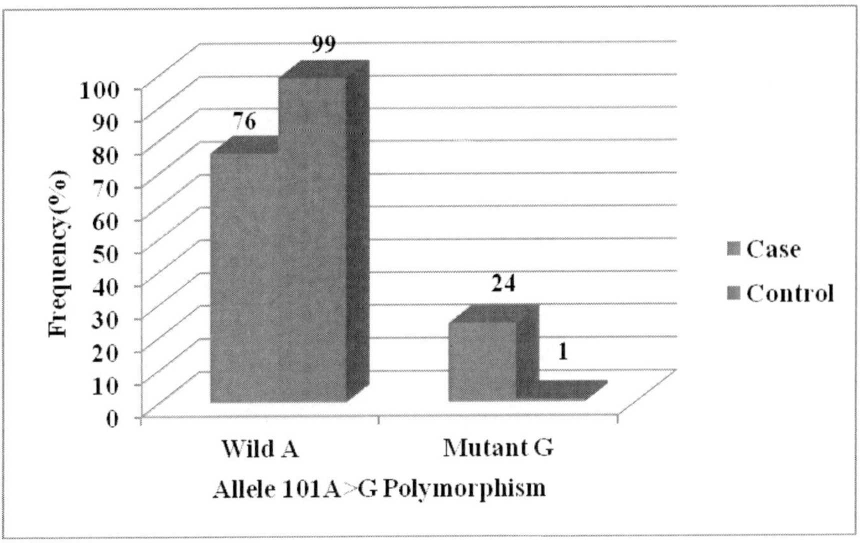

Figure 5.9. Allele frequency of 101A>G polymorphism.

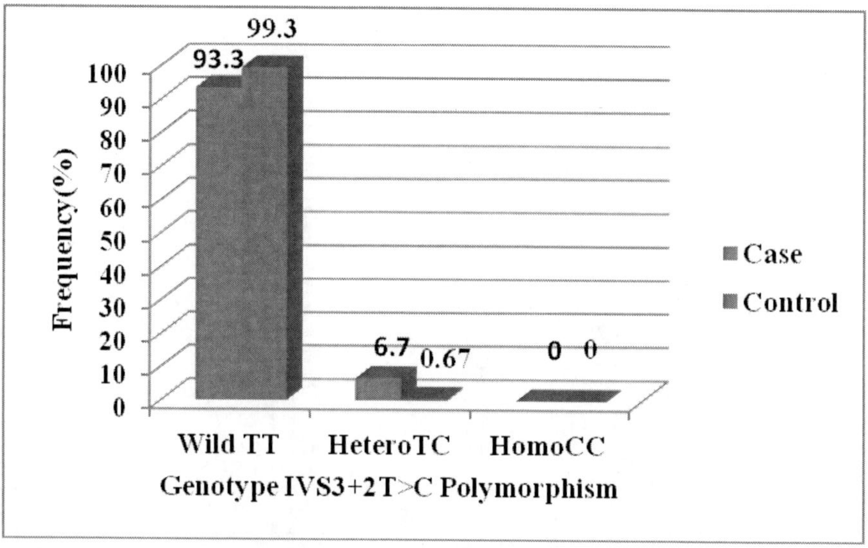

Figure 5.10. Genotype frequency of 1VS3+2T>C polymorphism.

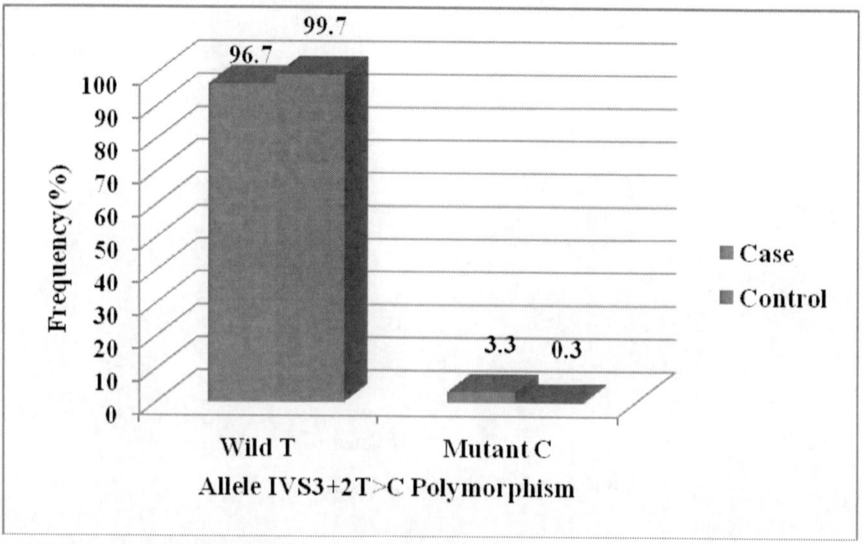

Figure 5.11. Allele frequency of IVS3+2T>C polymorphism.

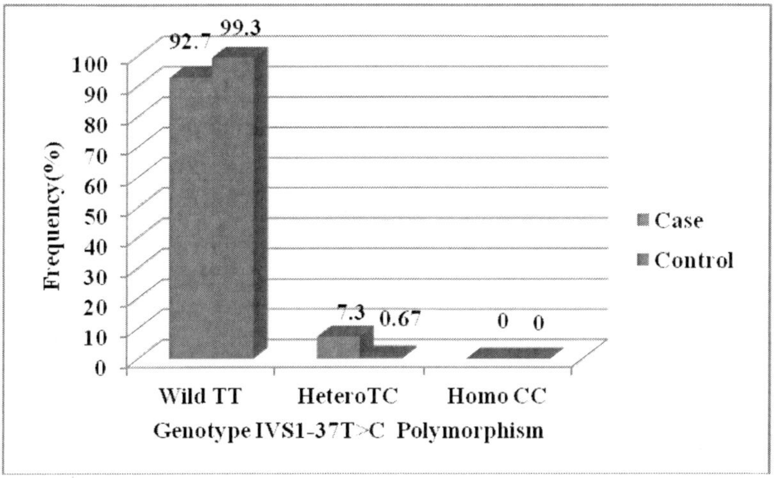

Figure 5.12. Genotype frequency of 1VS1-37T>C polymorphism.

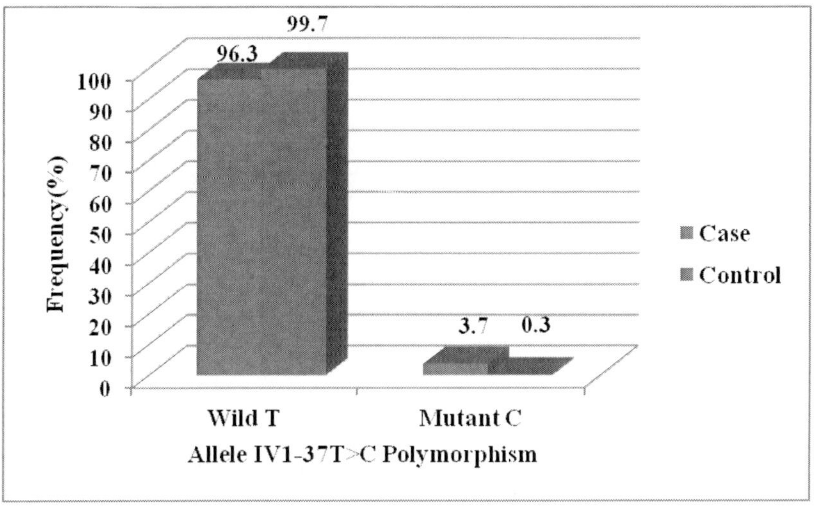

Figure 5.13. Allele frequency of IVS1-37T>C polymorphism.

5.3.1. Mutation ΔF508

Among 150 cases, 91.3% (137) were of wild type genotype, 8.7% (13) were of heterozygous and no homozygous mutation were found. Similarly in 150 controls, 98% (147) were of wild type genotype, 1.9% (3) were of heterozygous and no homozygous mutation were found. Heterozygous mutation was found to be associated with four times increased risk of TCP in comparison to Control (p=0.020; OR=4.65). The results are shown in Figure 5.14. A significant difference was observed between two groups OR: 4.65, 95%CI: 1.29-16.674, p-value: 0.020. The mutant allele frequency was found 4.3 (13) in cases as compared to 1% (3) controls. The results are shown in Figure 5.15. A significant association was observed in the frequency distribution of mutant allele with 4.4 times risk of disease with OR: 4.4, 95% CI 1.26-15.906, p-value 0.022.

5.3.2. Mutation G551D

Among 150 cases, 94% (141) were of wild type genotype, 6(9) were of heterozygous and no homozygous mutation was found. Similarly in 150 controls, 97.3% (146) were of wild type genotype, 2.7% (4) were of heterozygous and no homozygous were found. The results are shown in Figure 5.16. The odds ratio was (OR: 2.3, 95%CI: 0.70-7.74, p-value: 0.25). The wild type and mutant allele was found 97% (291) and 3% (9) in cases, respectively. In controls wild type and mutant allele was found 98.6% (296) and 1.3% (4) respectively. The results are shown in Figure 5.17. However, no association was observed between genotype and allele frequency. The results are shown in Table 5.5.

5.3.3. Mutation G542X

Among 150 cases, 93.3% (140) were of wild type genotype, 6.7 (10) were of heterozygous and no homozygous mutation was found. Similarly in 150 controls, 98% (147) were of wild type genotype, 2% (3) were of heterozygous and no homozygous were found. The results are shown in Figure 5.18. The odds ratio was (OR: 3.5, 95%CI: 0.94-12.986, p-value: 0.085). The wild type and mutant allele was found 97% (290) and 3.3% (10) in cases, respectively. In controls wild type and mutant allele was found 99% (297) and 1% (3), respectively. The results are shown in Figure 5.19. The risk was observed three times but no association was found between genotype and allele frequency. The results are shown in Table 5.5.

5.3.4. Mutation R117H

Among 150 cases, 98.6% (148) were of wild type genotype, 1.33 (2) were of heterozygous and no homozygous mutation was found. Similarly in 150 controls, 99.3% (149) were of wild type genotype, 0.66% (1) were of heterozygous and no homozygous mutation was found. The results are shown in Figure 5.20. The odds ratio was (OR: 1.3, 95%CI: 0.597-2.98, p-value: 1.0). The wild type and mutant allele was found 99.3% (298) and 0.66% (2) in cases respectively. In controls wild type and mutant allele was found 99.6% (299) and 0.33% (1), respectively. The results are shown in Figure 5.21. No association was found between genotype and allele frequency. The results are shown in Table 5.5.

5.3.5. Polymorphism S549N

Among 150 cases, 98% (147) were of wild type genotype, 2% (03) were of heterozygous and no homozygous mutation was found. Similarly in 150 controls, 99.3% (149) were of wild type genotype, 0.66% (01) were of heterozygous and no homozygous mutation was found. The results are shown in Figure 5.22. The odds ratio was OR: 1.5, 95%CI: 0.847-2.690, p-value: 0.6225. The wild type and mutant allele was found 99% (297) and 1% (3) in cases respectively. In controls wild type and mutant allele was found 99.6% (299) and 0.33% (1), respectively. The results are shown in Figure 5.23. No association was found between genotype and allele frequency. The results are shown in Table 5.5.

5.3.6. Polymorphism IVS8-T_n Tract (5T, 7T, 9T)

The analysis was carried out in 150 cases in which 92% (132) were of wild type genotype, 7.3% (11) were heterozygous and 0.66% (1) was homozygous. Similarly in controls 98% (147) were of wild type genotype, 2% (3) were heterozygous and no homozygous mutation was found. Heterozygous (7T/5T, 9T/5T) was found to be associated with four times risk of CP in comparison to control. A significant association was observed between two groups with OR: 3.90 95% CI: 1.067-14.301, P-0.003. The results are shown in Figure 5.24. The mutant allele frequency 5T was found 8.6% (13) in cases as compared to 1% (3) in controls. The results are shown in Figure 5.25. A significant association was found in the frequency distribution of mutant allele with OR: 1.9 95% CI (1.60-2.246) P-0.003. The results are shown in Table 5.5.

Table 5.5. Genotype and Allele Frequency of CFTR gene

Polymorphism	Type	TCP (n=150) %	Cont (n=150) %	OR (95% CI) p-value
ΔF508 Genotypes	Wild (FF)	137 (91.3)	147 (98)	Reference
	Heterozygous (FT)	13 (8.7)	03 (1.9)	4.65 (1.29-16.67)0.020*
ΔF508 Alleles	Wild allele (F)	287 (95.7)	297 (99)	Reference
	Mutant allele (T)	13 (4.3)	3 (1)	4.4 (1.26-15.906) 0.022*
G542X Genotypes	Wild (GG)	140 (93.3)	147 (98)	Reference
	Heterozygous (GT)	10 (6.7)	3 (2)	3.5 (0.94-12.98)0.085
G542X Alleles	Wild allele (G)	290 (97)	297 (99)	Reference
	Mutant allele (T)	10 (3.3)	3 (1)	3.4 (0.929-12.53) 0.0925
G551D Genotypes	Wild (GG)	141 (94)	146 (97.3)	Reference
	Heterozygous (GA)	9(6)	4 (2.7)	2.3(0.70-7.74)0.25
G551D Alleles	Wild allele (G)	291 (97)	296 (98.6)	Reference
	Mutant allele (A)	9 (3)	4(1.3)	2.28(0.69-7.51) 0.26
R117H Genotypes	Wild (RR)	148(98.6)	149 (99.3)	Reference
	Heterozygous (RH)	2 (1.33)	1 (0.66)	1.3 (0.597-2.98)1.0
R117H Alleles	Wild allele (R)	298 (99.3)	299 (99.6)	Reference
	Mutant allele (H)	2 (0.66)	1 (0.33)	1.3 (0.597-2.98) 1.0
S549N Genotypes	Wild (GG)	147 (98)	149 (99.3)	Reference
	Heterozygous (GA)	03 (2)	01 (0.66)	1.5 (0.847-2.690) 0.6225
S549N Alleles	Wild allele (G)	297 (99)	299 (99.6)	Reference
	Heterozygous (A)	3 (1)	1 (0.3)	1.5 (0.849-2.666) 0.623
IVS8-T_n Genotypes	Wild Type (7T/7T,9T/7T,9T/9T)	138 (92)	147 (98)	Reference
	Heterozygous (7T/5T, 9T/5T)	11 (7.3)	03 (2)	3.90 (1.067-14.301)0.03*
	Mutant (5T/5T)	01 (0.66)	0	
IVS8-T_n Alleles	Wild allele (7T,9T)	284 (94.6)	297 (99)	Reference
	Mutant allele (5T)	13 (8.6)	03 (1)	1.9 (1.60-2.246) 0.003*

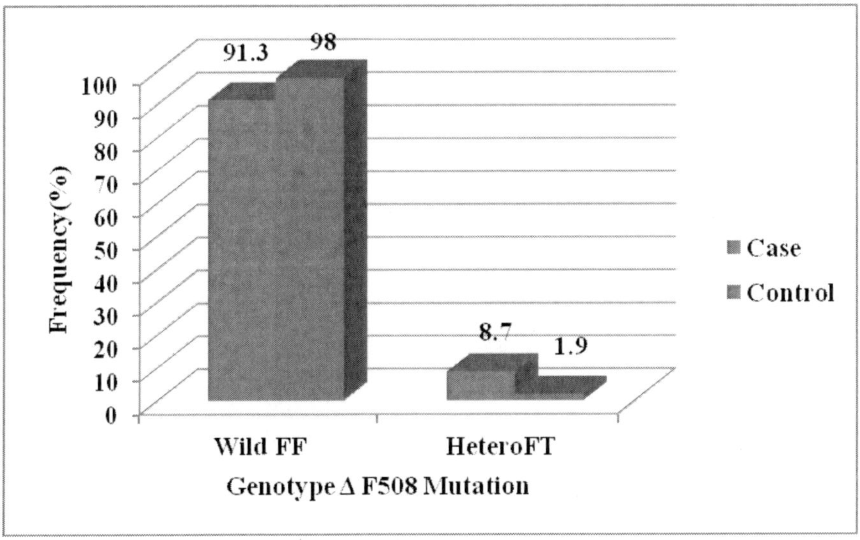

Figure 5.14. Genotype frequency of ΔF508 mutation.

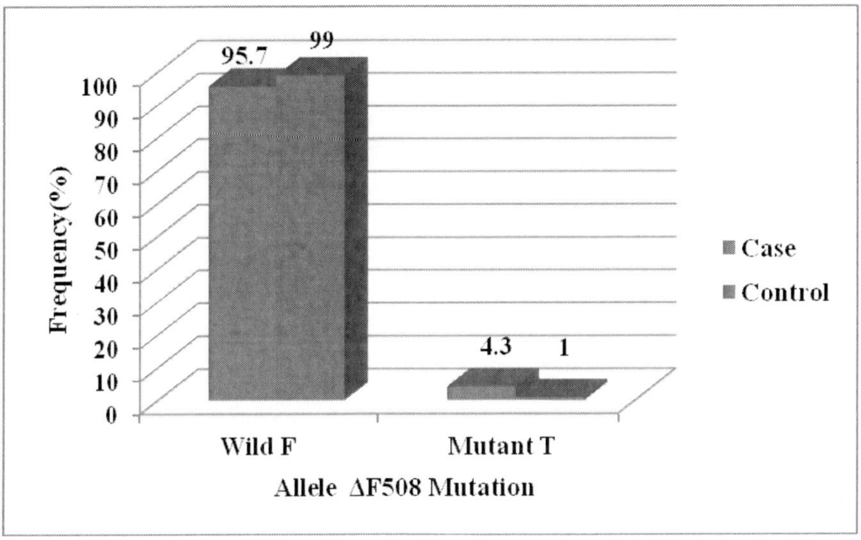

Figure 5.15. Allele frequency of ΔF508 mutation.

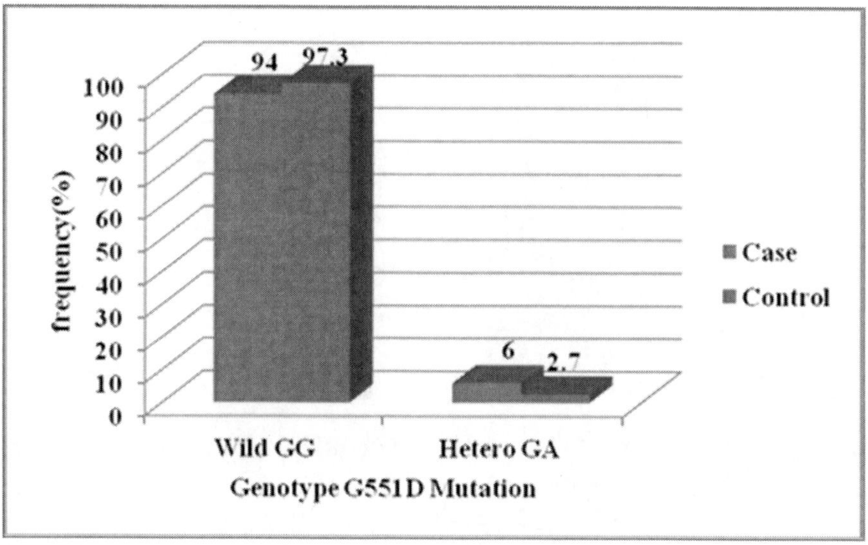

Figure 5.16. Genotype frequency of G551D mutation.

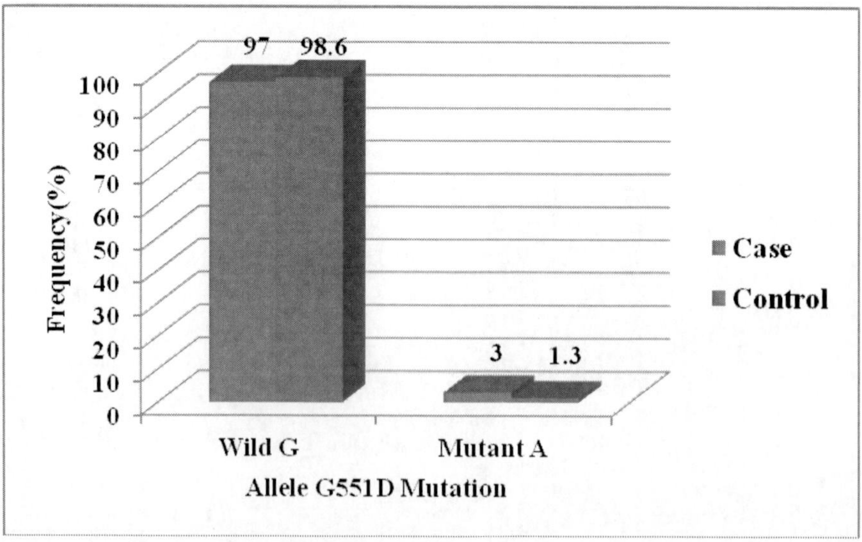

Figure 5.17. Allele frequency of G551D mutation.

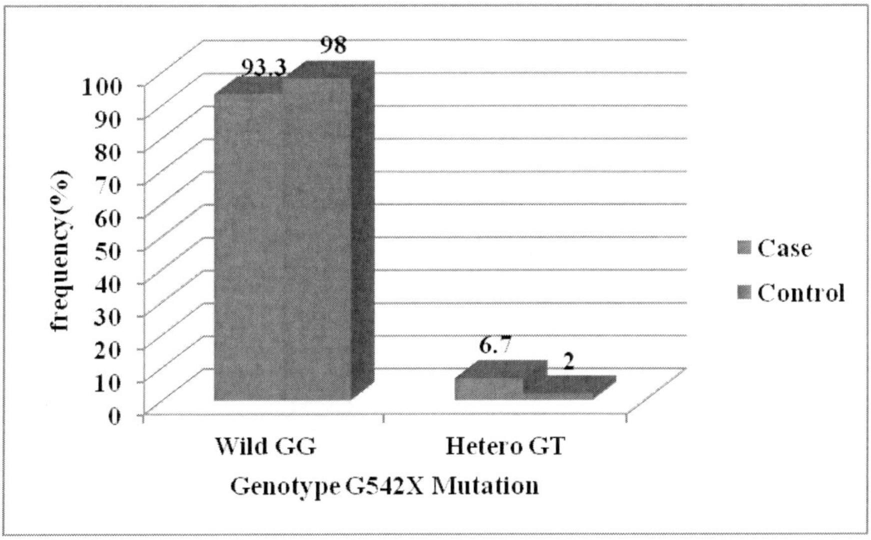

Figure 5.18. Genotype frequency of G542X mutation.

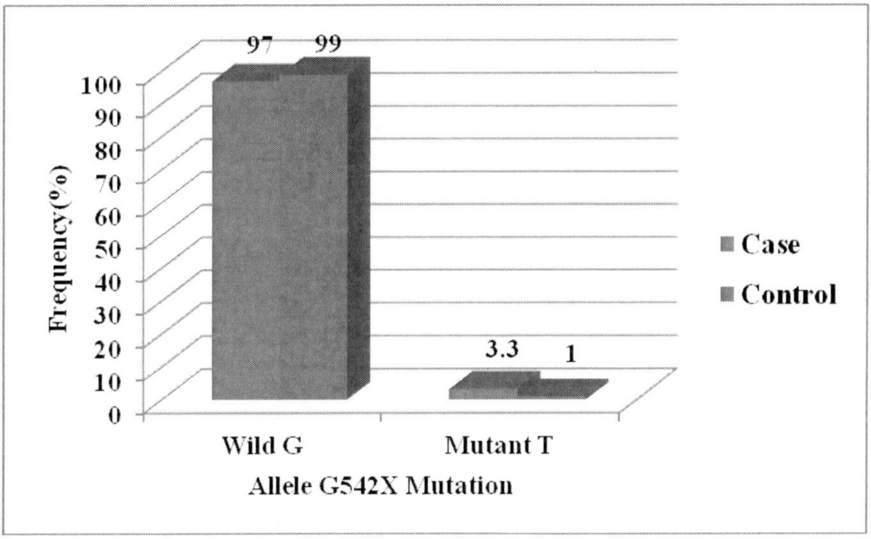

Figure 5.19. Allele frequency of G542X mutation.

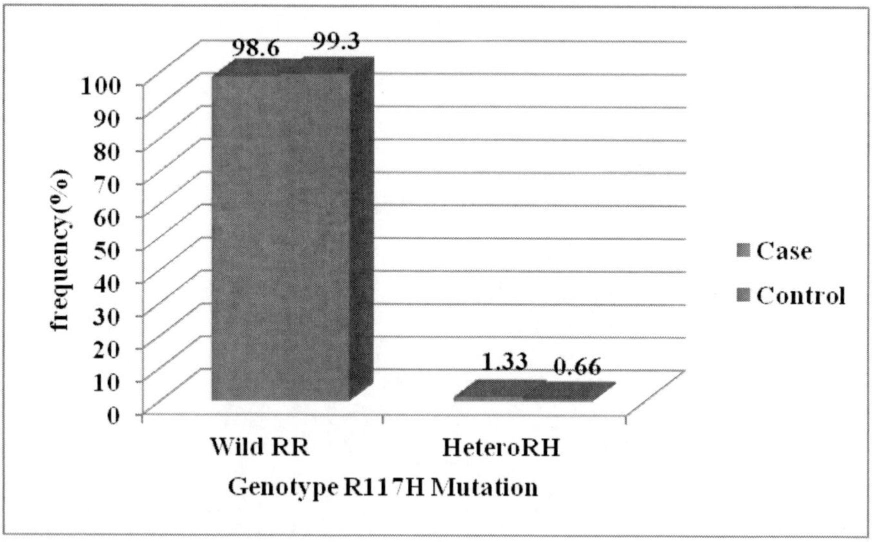

Figure 5.20. Genotype frequency of R117H mutation.

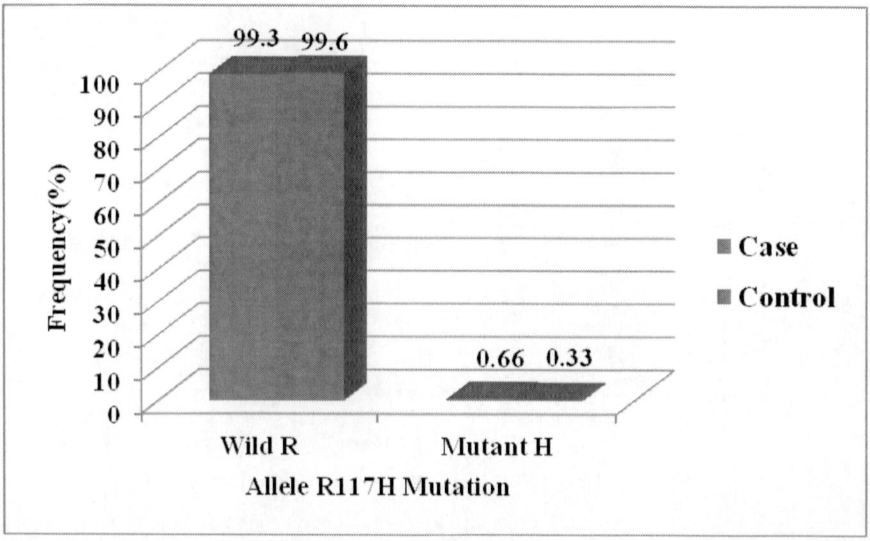

Figure 5.21. Allele frequency of R117H mutation.

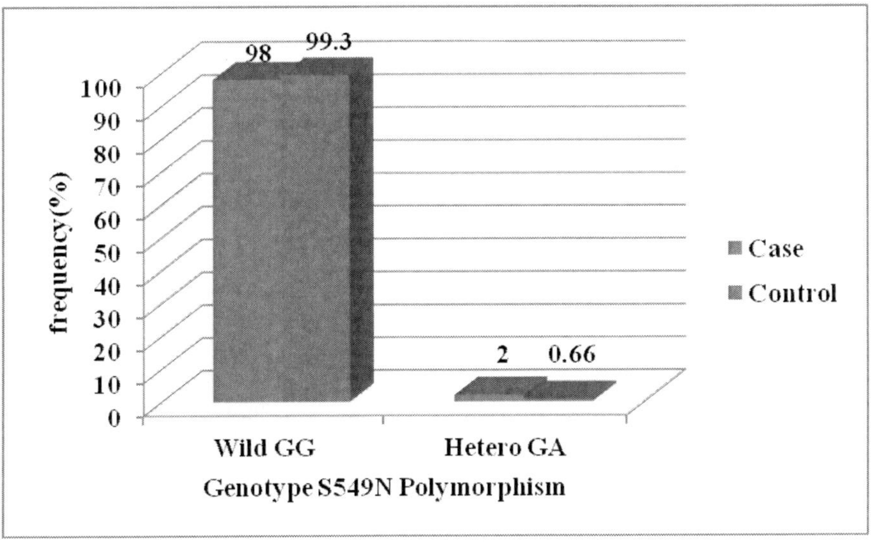

Figure 5.22. Genotype frequency of S549N polymorphism.

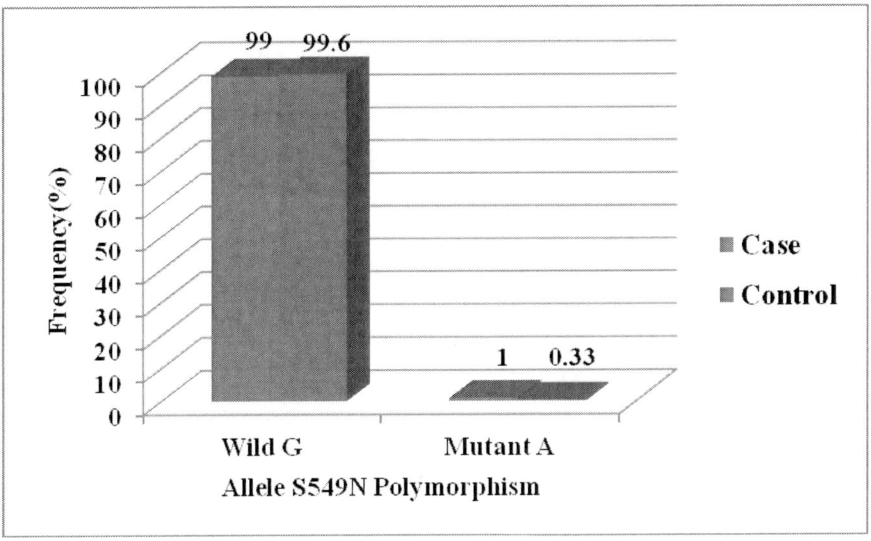

Figure 5.23. Allele frequency of S549N polymorphism.

5.4. Genotype and Allele Frequency of CTSB Gene

The genotype and allele frequency of CTSB gene was carried out in 150 cases of TCP and 150 cases of controls. All the samples were tested for one polymorphism, Leu26Val, by PCR-RFLP method described by Mahurkar et al. 2006.

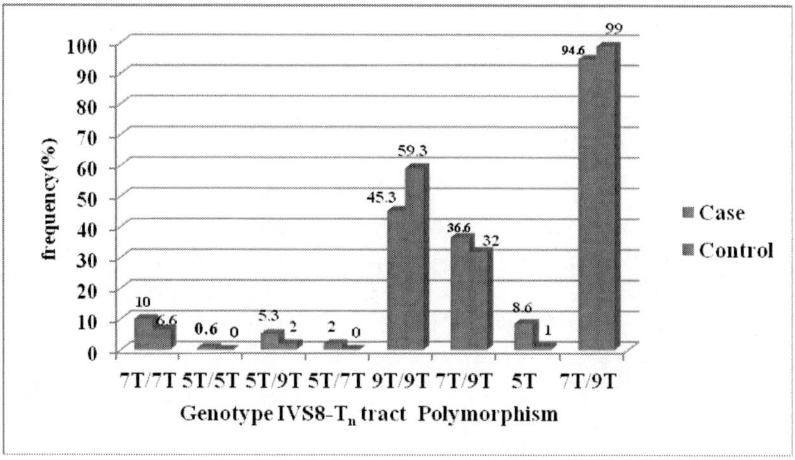

Figure 5.24. Genotype frequency of IVS8-T_n tract polymorphism.

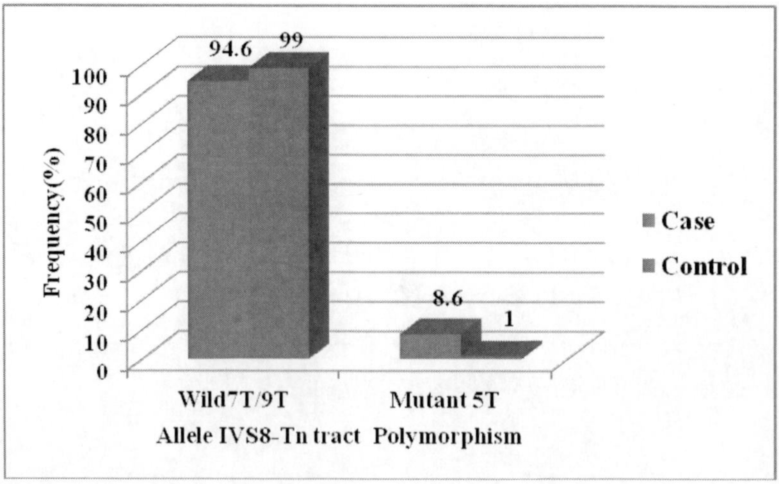

Figure 5.25. Allele frequency of IVS8-T_n tract polymorphism.

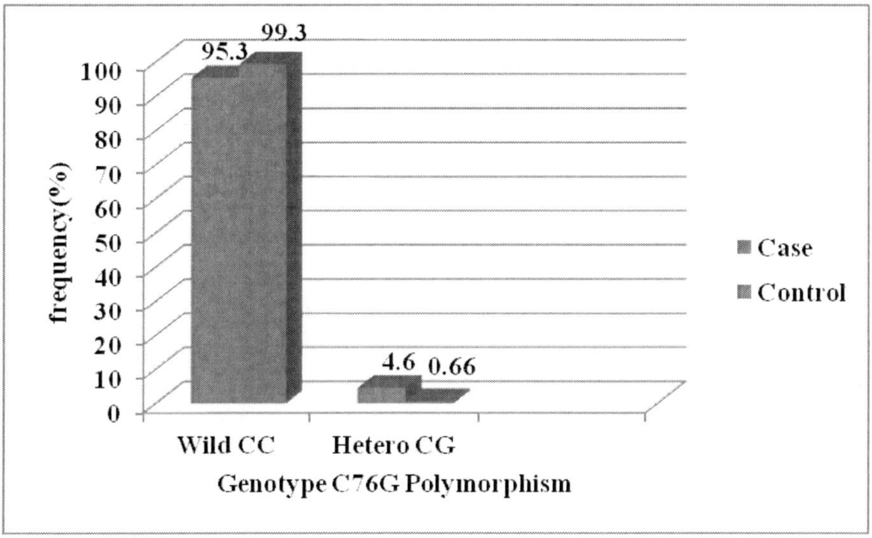

Figure 5.26. Genotype frequency of C76G polymorphism.

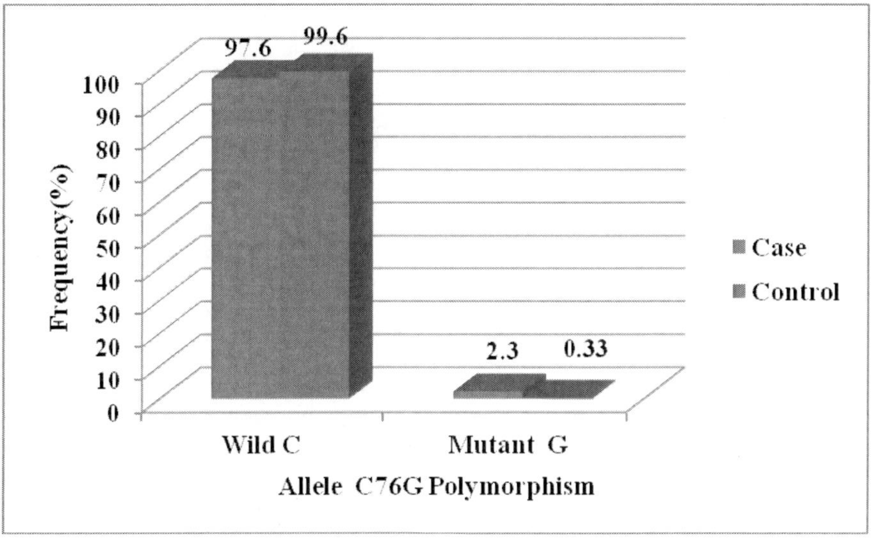

Figure 5.27. Allele frequency of C76G polymorphism.

5.4.1. Leu26Val (C76G) Polymorphism

Among 150 cases, 95.3% (143) were of wild type genotype, 4.6 % (7) were of heterozygous and no homozygous mutation was found. Similarly in 150 controls, 99.3% (149) were of wild type genotype, 0.66% (1) were of heterozygous and no homozygous mutation was found. The results are shown in Figure 5.26. The odds ratio was (OR: 1.7, 95%CI: 1.341-2.381, p-value: 0.667). The wild type and mutant allele was found 97.6% (293) and 2.3% (7) in cases, respectively. In controls wild type and mutant allele was found 99.6% (299) and 0.33% (1), respectively. The results are shown in Figure 5.27. No association of genotype and allele frequency was observed in TCP cases. The results are shown in Table 5.6.

Table 5.6. Genotype and Allele Frequency of C76G Polymorphism

Polymorphisms	Type	TCP (n=150) (%)	Cont (n=150) (%)	OR (95% CI) p-value
C76G Genotypes	Wild (CC)	143(95.3)	149(99.3)	Reference
	Heterozygous (CG)	7(4.6)	1(0.66)	1.7(1.341-2.381) 0.667
C76G Alleles	Wild allele (C)	293(97.6)	299(99.6)	Reference
	Mutant allele (G)	7(2.3)	1(0.33)	1.7 (1.344-2.326) 0.0685

5.5. Genotype and Allele Frequency of MTHFR Gene

The genotype and allele frequency of MTHFR gene was carried out in 150 cases of TCP and 150 cases of controls. All the samples were tested for one polymorphism C677T by PCR-RFLP method described by *Frosst et al. 1995.*

5.5.1. C677T Polymorphism

Among 150 cases, 57.3% (86) were of wild type genotype, 32.6% (49) were of heterozygous and 10% (15) were of homozygous. Similarly in 150 controls, 90.6% (136) were of wild type genotype, 8% (12) were of heterozygous and 1.3% (2) were of homozygous. Heterozygous CT associated with two times risk of disease. The results are shown in Figure 5.28. The odds ratio was OR: 2.7, 95%CI: 1.686-2.550, p-value: 0.001. The wild type and mutant allele was found 73.6% (221) and 26.3% (79) in cases respectively. In controls wild type and mutant allele was found 94.6% (284) and 6% (18) respectively. The results are shown in Figure 5.29. A significant association was observed between genotype and allele frequency. The results are shown in Table 5.7.

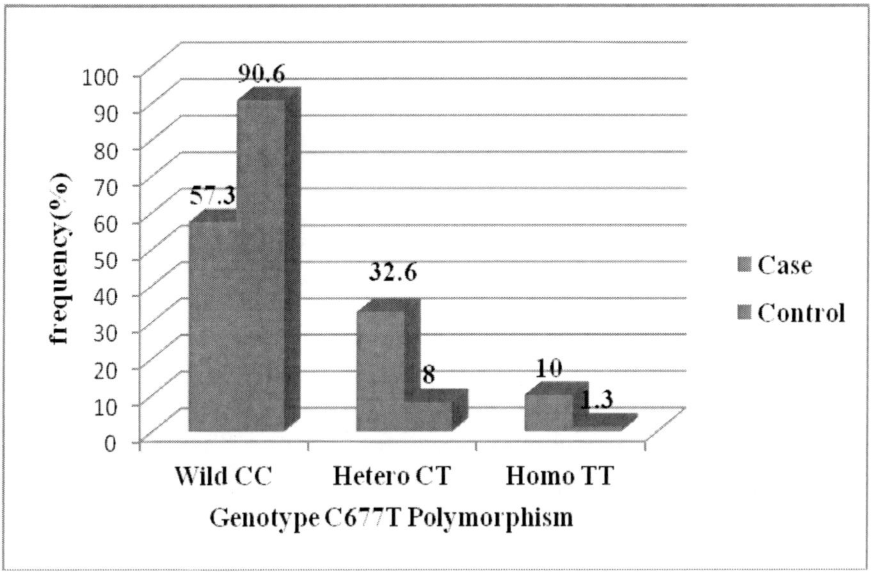

Figure 5.28. Genotype frequency of C677T polymorphism.

Table 5.7. Genotype and allele Frequency of C677T Polymorphism

Polymorphisms	Type	CP (n=150) (%)	Cont (n=150) (%)	OR (95% CI) p-value
C677T Genotypes	Wild (CC)	86(57.3)	136(90.6)	Reference
	Heterozygous (CT)	49(32.6)	12 (8)	2.7(1.686-2.550) 0.001
	Homozygous (TT)	15(10)	2 (1.3)	
C677T Alleles	Wild allele (C)	221(73.6)	284(94.6)	Reference
	Mutant allele (T)	79(26.3)	8(6)	1.9 (1.662-2.173) 0.001

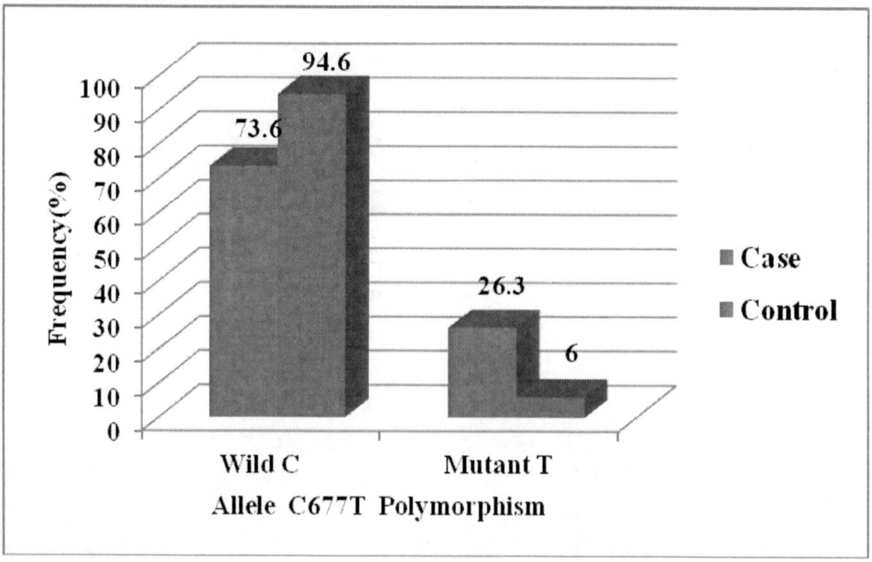

Figure 5.29. Allele frequency of C677T polymorphism.

5.6. Genotype and Allele Frequency of ACE Gene

The genotype and allele frequency of ACE gene was carried out in 150 cases of TCP and 150 cases of controls. All the samples were tested for ACE Insertion / Deletion Polymorphisms by ARMS PCR method described by Berge et al. 1997.

5.6.1. ACEI / D Polymorphism

The observed DD genotype frequency among cases and control groups was 28 % (42), while that of in the control group was 31.3 (47). No significant association was observed between ACE gene polymorphism with Chronic Pancreatitis (p=0.671, OR=0.927, 95% CI: 0.698–1.233). The results are shown in Figure 5.30. The genotype frequency of ID was found almost similar frequency in case and control 33.3% and 31.3%, respectively, and no association was observed between the groups. p=1.01 95% CI 0.779-1.320 OR 1.0. The results are shown in Table 5.8. The frequency of I allele was higher in both the cases 55.3% (166) and the controls 53% (159) (p=0.623, OR= 0.954,

95% CI: 0.811–1.121). No association was found between the groups. The results are shown in Figure 5.31.

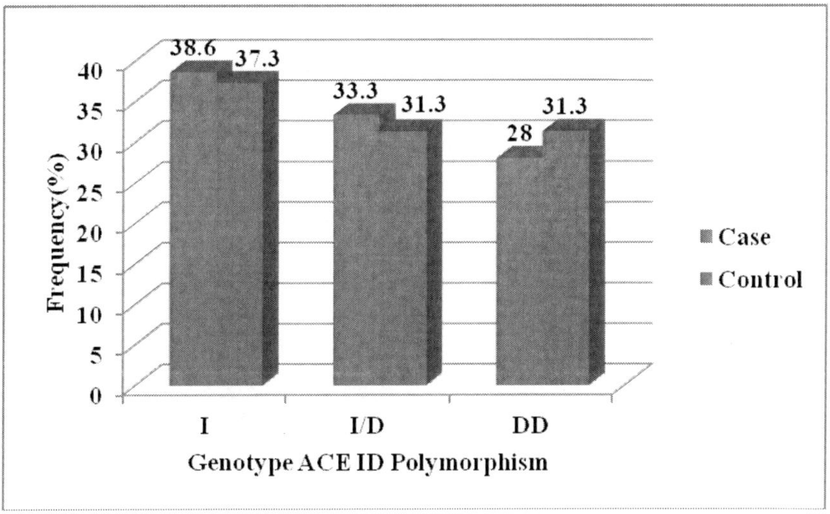

Figure 5.30. Genotype frequency of ACE polymorphism.

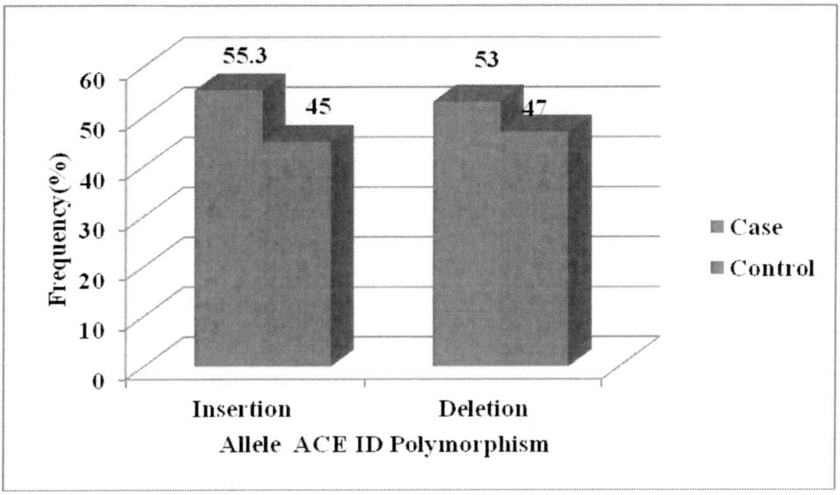

Figure 5.31. Allele frequency of ACE polymorphism.

Table 5.8. Genotype and allele Frequency of ACEID Polymorphism

Polymorphisms	Type	CP (n=150) (%)	Cont (n=150) (%)	OR (95% CI) p-value
ACE I/D Genotypes	Insertion (II)	58(38.6)	56(37.3)	Reference
	Insertion/ Deletion(ID)	50(33.3)	47(31.3)	1.01(0.779-1.320) 1.0
	Deletion (DD)	42(28)	47(31.3)	0.927(0.6981.233) 0.671
ACE I/D Alleles	Insertion (I)	166(55.3)	159(53)	Reference
	Deletion (D)	134(45)	141(47)	0.954 (0.811-1.121)0.623

5.7. Genotype-Phenotype Correlation Between SPINK1 Gene Polymorphism and Tropical Chronic Pancreatitis (TCP)

In order to achieve secondary objective, mutants of *SPINK1* gene variants among cases were compared with wild type. Mutants were defined as those subjects which were found heterozygous for any of the three variants (polymorphism: N34S, IVS3+2T>C, and IVS1-37T>C) studied whereas; Wild type are those subjects which were homozygous for the wild type allele. Analysis of N34S carrier frequency after categorizing our study cohort in to groups by age showed interesting results. The < 20 yrs groups had a carrier frequency of 41.5 % (22 of 53) which is significantly higher than that of 36% (35 of 97) in the 20-60 years old group ($p<0.016$). We categorized the study cohort according to etiology and then compared the SPINK1 N34S positive and negative patients in each category as a function of various phenotypic markers.

5.7.1. Distribution of Various Clinical Parameters among Patients with Tropical Chronic Pancreatitis Based on N34S SPINK1 Polymorphism Status

The results of analysis of distribution of various clinical parameters like calcification, pain, diabetes and smoking among patients with TCP based on N34S SPINK1 polymorphism have been shown in the Table 5.9.

Table 5.9. N34S SPINK1 polymorphism with calcification

Tropical Chronic Pancreatitis (n=150)	Calcification		OR (95% CI) p-value
	Present	Absent	
Polymorphism positive	48	18	0.032 (0.1329-0.7704) 0.0161
Polymorphism Negative	75	9	Reference
Total	123	27	

The SPINK1N34S polymorphism was identified in 32% (48) cases with calcification and in 12% (18) of mutated patient where calcification was not present (OR: 0.032, 95%CI: 0.1329-0.7704) p-value: 0.0161). Calcification is a factor associated with N34S mutation showed similar trends suggested that mutation status directly related to the calcification. However, a significant difference between the polymorphism positive and polymorphism negative was observed between the two groups. The results are shown in Figure 5.32.

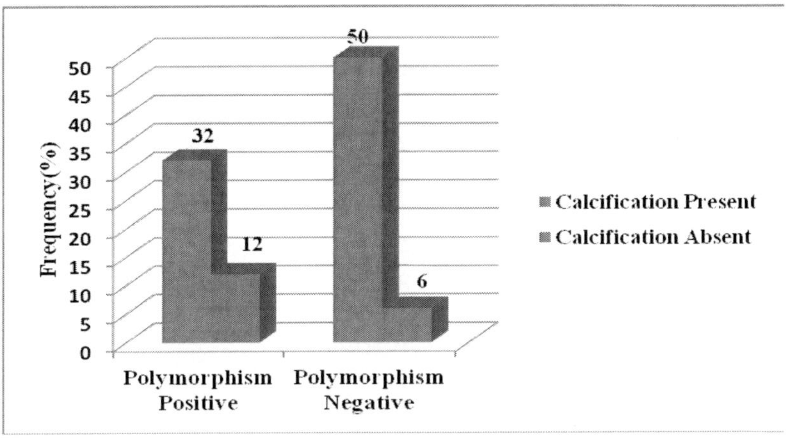

Figure 5.32. Distribution of mutated and negative SPINK1 N34S in calcification.

5.7.2. N34S SPINK1 Polymorphism with Pain

The analysis of status of N34S SPINK1 polymorphism with Pain among TCP cases and controls has been displayed in the Table 5.10.

Table 5.10. Analysis of status of N34S SPINK1 polymorphism with Pain among TCP cases and controls

Tropical Chronic Pancreatitis (n=150)	Pain			p-value
	Mild	Moderate	Severe	
Polymorphism Positive	12	30	46	0.811
Polymorphism Negative	18	25	19	
Total	30	55	65	

The SPINK1N34S polymorphism was identified in 8% (12) cases with mild intermittent pain with 20% (30) had moderate constant pain as compared with SPINK1 N34S polymorphism negative 12% (18) of mild and 16.6% (25) had moderate pain respectively with no significant association of patients with mild to moderate pain with N34S mutation, this might another factor predominant in disease progression. When compared the mutated SPINK1 N34S mutation in patients with mild pain and compared to severe constant pain with frequency of 30.6% (46). However no significant association between two groups with p-value 0.811. The results are shown in Figure 5.33.

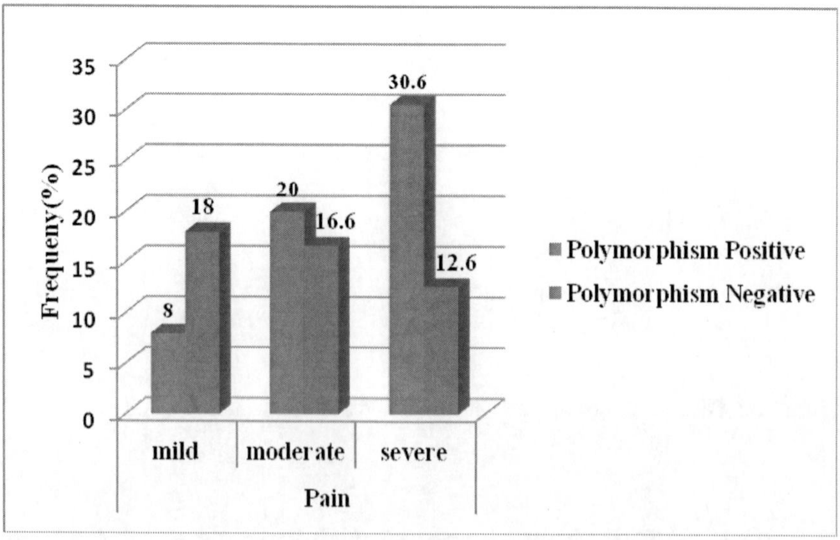

Figure 5.33. Distribution of mutated and negative SPINK1 N34S with pain.

5.7.3. N34S SPINK1 Polymorphism with Diabetes

The analysis of status of N34S SPINK1 polymorphism with diabetes among TCP cases and controls has been displayed in the Table 5.11.

Table 5.11. Analysis of status of N34S SPINK1 polymorphism with diabetes among TCP cases and controls

Tropical Chronic Pancreatitis (n=150)	Diabetes	Non-diabetic	OR (95% CI) p-value
Polymorphism Positive	39	27	3.049 (1.558-5.967) 0.001
Polymorphism Negative	27	57	Reference
Total	66	84	

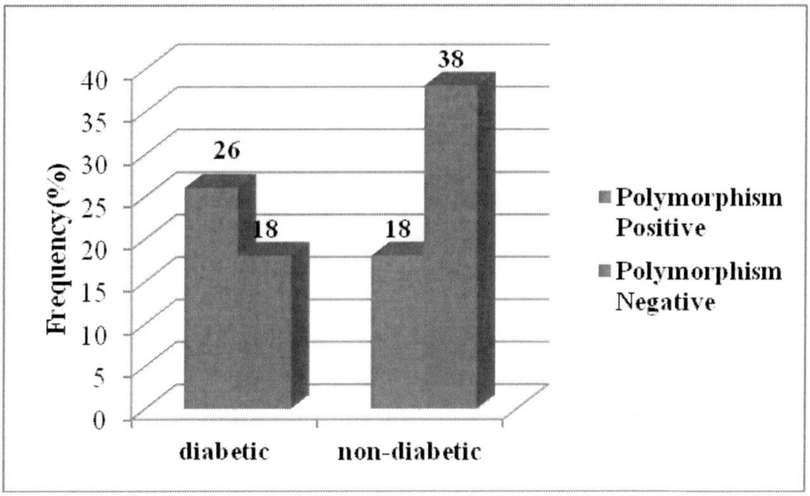

Figure 5.34. Distribution of mutated and negative SPINK1 N34S polymorphism with diabetes.

Diabetes mellitus as a feature of pancreatic endocrine insufficiency was prevalent in 26% (39) of chronic pancreatitis patients with diabetes as predisposing factors with mutated SPINK1 N34S polymorphism as compared to 18% (27) of non-diabetic patients. A comparison of SPINK1 polymorphism frequency in TCP patients with diabetes and without diabetes show the trend of disease severity suggesting that mutation status is directly related to the presentation of diabetes. Negative SPINK1 N34S polymorphism in diabetes was found 18% (27) as compared to non-diabetic 38% (57). On comparing two parameters we found significant association and three times the risk of disease with odds ratio OR: 3.049, 95%CI 1.558-5.967 p-value 0.001. The results are shown in Figure 5.34. This may be due to additional environmental or genetic factors associated with N34S mutation. A significant association was observed between N34S mutation and diabetes.

5.7.4. N34S SPINK1 Polymorphism with Smoking

The analysis of status of N34S SPINK1 polymorphism with smoking among TCP cases and controls has been displayed in the Table 5.12.

Table 5.12. Analysis of status of N34S SPINK1 polymorphism with smoking

Tropical Chronic Pancreatitis (n=150)	Smoking		OR (95% CI) p-value
	Smoker	Non-smoker	
Polymorphism positive	34	32	1.18 (0.9431-3.499) 0.096
Polymorphism Negative	31	53	Reference
Total	85	65	

Prevalence of N34S SPINK1 mutation 22.6% (34) in patients with smoker was similar in patients with non-smoker 32(21.3%). Therefore, no association was observed between N34S polymorphism and smoking OR: 1.18, 95%CI 0.9431-3.499 p-value 0.096. This may be due to other factors associated with other TCP groups as the prevalence of N34S mutation was comparable in both the groups. The negative N34S mutation prevalence in smoker 20.6% as compared to non-smoker 35.3% showed variability in the mutation status with different groups. The results are shown in Figure 5.35.

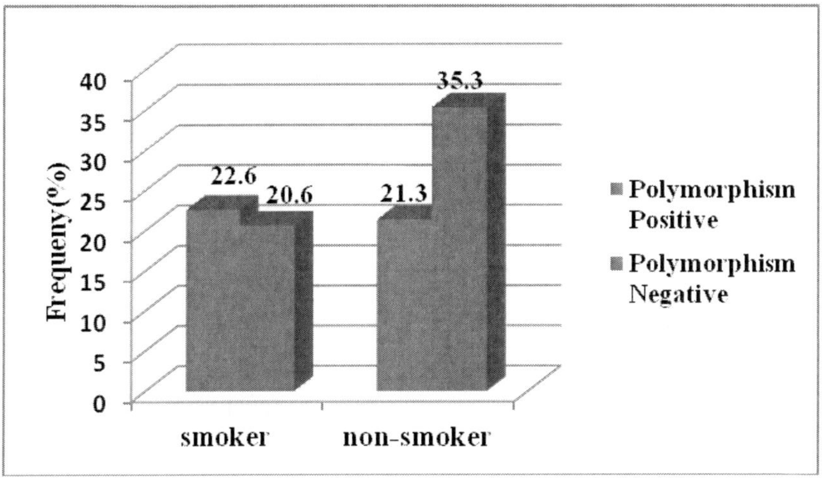

Figure 5.35. Distribution of mutated and negative SPINK1 N34S muation with smoking.

5.8. Combined Effect of SPINK1 Gene Variants on Phenotypes

The categorization of various phenotypic features in patients with and without SPINK1 mutations carriers vs. non-carriers was comparable. It is now considered that SPINK1 gene mutation play a modifier role in function of various phenotypic features of TCP. So to differentiate the role of other biochemical parameter with SPINK1 polymorphism, the clinical and biochemical findings of TCP and SPINK1 carriers and non-carriers are summarized in Table 5.13.

In 150 TCP patients, the carrier's frequency of SPINK1 mutations was 88 (58.6%) compared to the non-carriers frequency 62 (41.3%). The prevalence of mutations was higher in more than 50% of patients and was found to be strongly associated with TCP. The data obtained after analysis of different lipid profiles (triglycerides, total cholesterol, HDL, LDL and VLDL) indicated that the content of serum high-density lipoprotein (HDL) was significant (p=0.002) as it reflected almost 50% lower value in carriers as compared to the non-carriers. In contrast, the level of VLDL was significantly higher in the carriers as compared to the non-carriers. However the levels of serum triglyceride, total cholesterol and LDL demonstrated no significant association between these two groups. Among the two key serum enzymes tested, the carriers displayed very high level of serum amylase as compared to the non-carriers. In contrast, the level of serum lipase (p=0.012) was found to be higher in the non-carriers as compared to the non-carriers group. Taken together, it appears that the levels of certain biochemical indices such as HDL and VLDL as well as the activities of serum amylase possess significant association with TCP.

Table 5.13. Demographic and clinical profiles of 150 TCP cases (carriers vs. non-carriers) screened for SPINK1 gene

Characteristics	Carriers (88)	Non carriers (62)	p-value
Age in months (M±SD)	33.9±11.7	32.3±11.6	0.395
Weight in kg (M± SD)	56.0±13.3	52.2±12.8	0.082
BMI(M ±SD)	21.2±4.6	20.1±4.5	0.132
FBS (M±SD)	56.2±102.6	48.2±103.8	0.567
PPBS (M±SD)	153.6±79.3	168.9±68.5	0.210
HbA1C(M±SD)	5.93±1.7	5.23±1.5	0.225
Triglyceride(M±SD)	118.2±92.0	116.3±59.56	0.883
Total Cholesterol	156.1±51.29	162±49.3	0.381
HDL-cholesterol	35.8±8.82	76.3±9.86	0.002*
LDL-cholesterol	86.2±32.2	88.8±28.7	0.432
VLDL-cholesterol	26.9±12.41	17.5±7.77	0.012*
Serum Amylase	1023±488.8	727.7±480	0.013*
Serum Lipase	732.40±452.2	888.9±420	0.112
Serum Calcium	8.9±1.2	9.11±1.09	0.226

Each value has been expressed as Mean's. (* Significant Association found)

5.8.1. SPINK1 Gene Carriers and Non-carriers Polymorphism Status with Calcification

The analysis of association of SPINK1 polymorphism (N34S, IVS3+2T>C and IVS1-37T>C) with calcification among TCP carriers and non-carriers has been displayed in the Table 5.14.

The carrier SPINK1 polymorphism was identified in 38% (57) of TCP patients has calcification and 13.3% (20) with absence of calcification. The most similar trend was observed in non-carriers with calcification and frequency was found 34% (51) OR: 0.590, 95%CI: 0.602-2.510, p-value:

1.229. However, no significant difference between the frequencies was observed between the two groups. The data are shown in Figure 5.36.

Table 5.14. Analysis of association of SPINK1 polymorphism with calcification among TCP carriers and non-carriers

Tropical Chronic Pancreatitis (n=150)	Calcification		OR (95% CI) p-value
	present	absent	
Carriers SPINK1 polymorphism	57	20	0.590 (0.602-2.510) 1.229
Non-carriers	51	22	
Total	108	42	

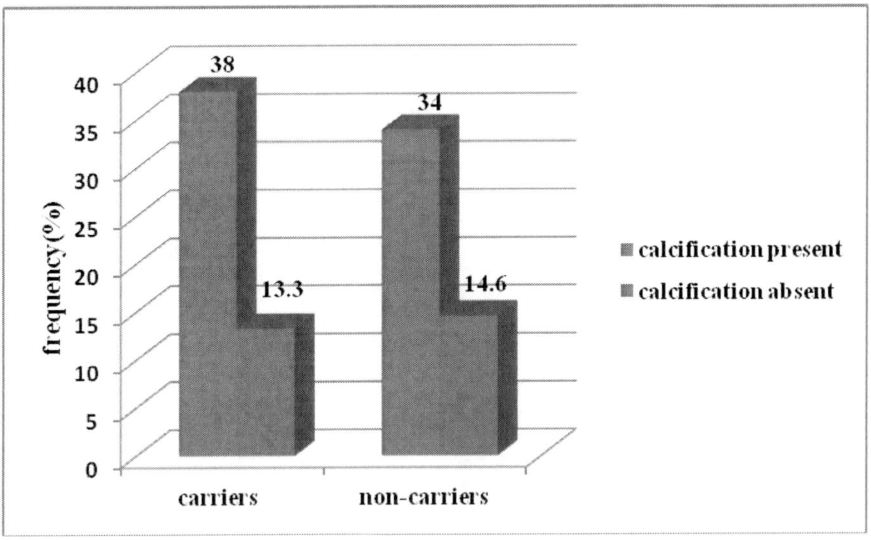

Figure 5.36. Distribution of carriers and non-carrier SPINK1 polymorphism with calcification.

5.8.2. SPINK1 Polymorphism Carrier Status with Pain

The analysis of SPINK1 polymorphism carrier status with pain are shown in Table 5.15.

Table 5.15. Analysis of SPINK1 polymorphism carrier status with pain

Tropical Chronic Pancreatitis (n=150)	Pain			OR (95% CI) p-value
	Mild	Moderate	Severe	
Carriers SPINK1 polymorphism	5	15	42	0.026
Non-carriers	13	35	40	
Total	18	50	82	

The carrier SPINK1 polymorphism was identified in 3% (5), 10% (15) and 28% (42) of patients with mild, moderate and severe pain respectively. In the non-carriers the frequency of SPINK1 polymorphism was 26.6% (40), in severe, 8.6 % (13) in mild and 23.3% (35) in moderate pain was found. No significant association was obtained with pain and SPINK1 polymorphism with P-value 0.026. The results are shown in Figure 5.37. So the presentation and age of onset of pain with different decades had no association with SPINK1 polymorphism, there may be another factors associated with the type of pain which might mask the effect of other factors.

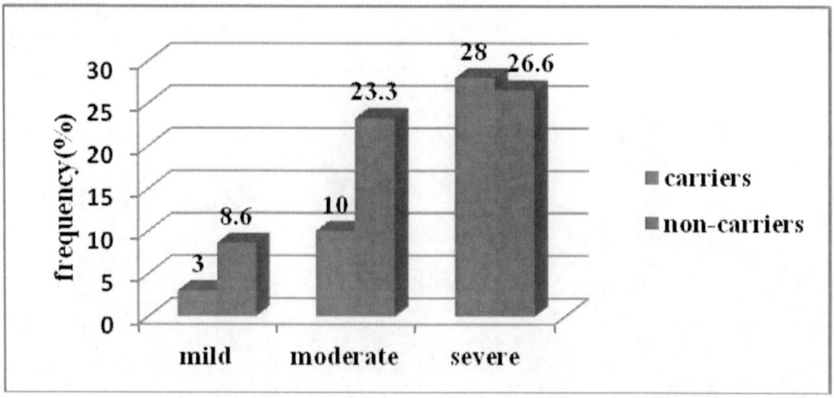

Figure 5.37. Distribution of carriers and non-carrier SPINK1 polymorphism with pain.

5.8.3. SPINK1 Polymorphism Carrier Status with Diabetes

The analysis of SPINK1 polymorphism carrier status with diabetes was shown in Table 5.16.

Table 5.16. Analysis of SPINK1 polymorphism carrier status with diabetes

Tropical Chronic Pancreatitis (n=150)	Diabetic	Non-diabetic	OR (95% CI) p-value
Carriers SPINK1Polymorphism	33	29	1.041 (0.763-1.419) 0.868
Non-carriers	45	43	
Total	78	72	

The carrier's frequency of SPINK1 polymorphism in TCP patients with diabetic was found 22% (33) compared to 19.3% (29) of non-diabetic. Non-carrier frequency of SPINK1 polymorphism was found 30% (45) in diabetic and 28.6% (43), in non-diabetic patients. However no association was found with SPINK1 carriers status and diabetes OR: 1.041, 95%CI: 0.763-1.419, p-value: 0.868). The results are shown in Figure 5.38. The exact relationship between the diabetes and TCP is not clear, although there is an overlap between the phenotypes and SPINK1 polymorphism carrier frequency.

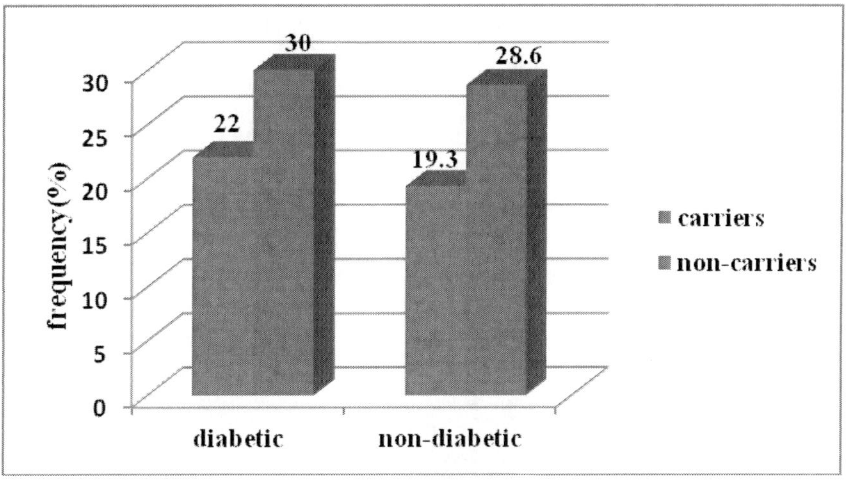

Figure 5.38. Distribution of carriers and non-carrierSPINK1 polymorphism with diabetes.

5.8.4. SPINK1 Polymorphism Carrier Status with Smoking

Analysis of association of SPINK1 polymorphism carrier status with smoking is shown in Table 5.17.

Table 5.17. Analysis of association of SPINK1 polymorphism carrier status with smoking

Tropical Chronic Pancreatitis(n=150)	Smoking		OR (95% CI) p-value
	Smoker	Non- smoker	
Carriers SPINK1 polymorphism	34	32	0.5748 (0.298-1.109) 0.135
Non-carriers	31	53	
Total	85	65	

The carrier frequency of SPINK1 gene polymorphism in smoker and non-smoker were 22.6% (34) and 21.3% (32) respectively. However 20.6% (31) of smokers and 35.3% (53) of were found negative for SPINK1 gene polymorphism. On analysis of SPINK1 and smokers no association was found with OR: 0.574, 95%CI: 0.298-1.109, p- value: 0.135**.** The results are shown in Figure 5.39.

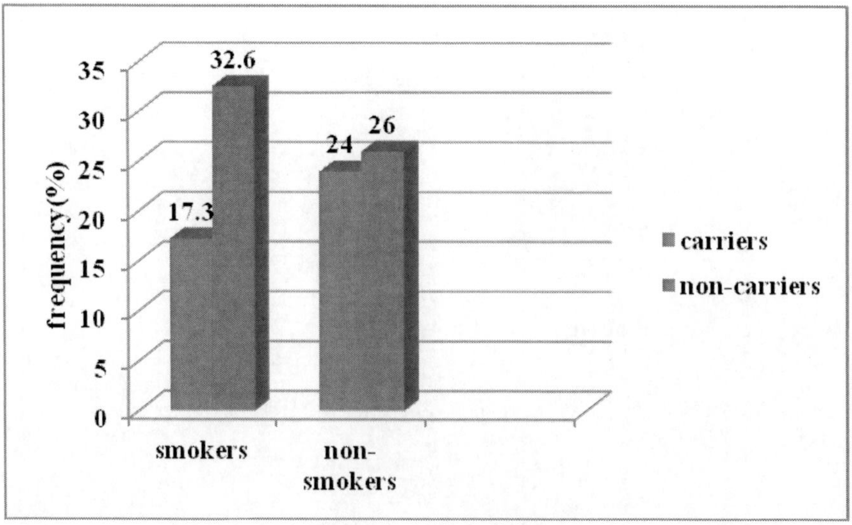

Figure 5.39. Distribution of carriers and non-carrierSPINK1 polymorphism with smoking.

5.9. Genotypic-Phenotypic Correlation between *CFTR* Gene Mutation and Tropical Chronic Pancreatitis (TCP)

The categorization of various phenotypic features in patients with and without CFTR mutations carriers vs. non-carriers was comparable. It is now considered that CFTR gene mutation play role in function of various phenotypic features. So to differentiate the role of other biochemical parameter with CFTR mutations, the clinical and biochemical findings of TCP and CFTR carriers and non-carriers are summarized in Table 5.18.

Table 5.18. Demographic and clinical profile of 150 Tropical Chronic Pancreatitis cases (carriers vs. non-carriers) screened for CFTR gene

Characteristics	Carriers (49)	Non carriers (101)	p-value
Age in months (M±SD)	36.1±11.63	31.8±11.5	0.036
Weight in kg (M± SD)	57±12.7	53.2±13.3	0.126
BMI(M ±SD)	21.2±4.21	20.5±4.77	0.309
FBS (M±SD)	117±58.5	96.3±48.6	0.022*
PPBS (M±SD)	174.3±86.16	153.3±68.4	0.109
HbA1C(M±SD)	5.29±1.7	5.65±1.65	0.223
Triglyceride(M±SD)	134.8±115.0	108.9±53.4	0.032*
Total Cholesterol (M±SD)	165.5±46.3	155.3±52.1	0.228
HDL-cholesterol (M±SD)	36.1±9.75	60.7±13.5	0.032
LDL-cholesterol	87.2±25.9	84.8±40.3	0.852
VLDL-cholesterol	28.3±11.2	22.3±13.4	0.296
Serum Amylase	607.2±540.0	722.7±465.7	0.179
Serum Lipase	825.4±639.1	569.5±443.1	0.035*
Serum Calcium	9.06±0.944	8.9±1.3	0.631

Mean±SD (Significant Association found)

In 150 TCP patients carrier's frequency of CFTR mutations was 32.6% (49) compared to non-carriers frequency 67.3% (101). The ΔF508 mutation was observed in 8.6% of CP patients as compared to other CFTR mutation comprises of frequency 24.6%. The data obtained after analysis of lipid profiles (triglycerides, total cholesterol, HDL, LDL and VLDL) indicated that the content of serum high-density lipoprotein (HDL) was significant (p=0.045) as it reflected almost 50% lower value in carriers as compared to the non-carriers. In contrast, the level of VLDL, Triglyceride was significantly higher in the carriers as compared to the non-carriers. However the levels of serum triglyceride, total cholesterol and LDL demonstrated no significant association between these groups.

Among the two key serum enzymes tested, the carriers displayed very high level of serum Lipase as compared to the non-carriers (p=0.035). In contrast, the level of serum amylase (p-0.179) was found to be higher in the non-carriers as compared to the carriers group. Taken together, it appears that the levels of certain biochemical indices such as HDL and triglyceride as well as the activities of serum lipase possess significant association with TCP.

5.9.1. CFTR Mutations Carrier Status with Calcification

Analysis of CFTR mutations carrier status with calcification is presented in the Table 5.19. The CFTR mutation carrier was identified in 26.6% (40) patients of calcification and 6.6% (10) with absence of calcification.

The non-carriers frequency of CFTR in calcification was observed 40% (60) as compared to patients with absence of calcification 26.6% (40) with OR: 2.6, 95%CI: 1.198-5.937, p-value: 0.016. A significant association was observed difference between CFTR mutation and calcification. The results are shown in Figure 5.40.

Table 5.19. Analysis of CFTR mutations carrier status with calcification is presented

Tropical Chronic Pancreatitis	**Calcification**		**OR (95% CI) p-value**
	present	**absent**	
CFTR mutation carriers	40	10	2.6(1.198-5.937) 0.016
Non-carriers	60	40	References
Total	100	50	

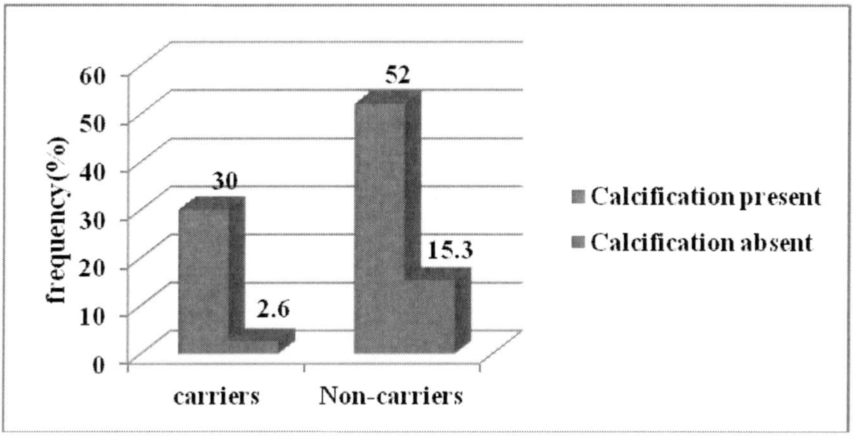

Figure 5.40. Distribution of carriers and non-carrier CFTR mutations with calcification.

5.9.2. CFTR Mutations Carrier Status with Pain

Analysis of CFTR mutations carrier status with pain is presented in the Table 5.20

Table 5.20. Analysis of CFTR mutations carrier status with pain

Tropical Chronic Pancreatitis (n=150)	Pain			OR (95% CI) p-value
	Mild	Moderate	Severe	
CFTR mutation carriers	4	13	32	
Non-carriers	14	37	50	0.182
Total	18	50	82	

The CFTR mutation carriers were identified in 2.6% (4) TCP patients with mild pain, 8.6% (13) moderate and 21.3% (32) of severe pain. Non-carriers frequency observed were 14 (9.3%), 37 (24.6%) and 50 (33.3%) in mild, moderate and severe pain, respectively. However no significant association was observed with CFTR mutation and pain with P-value 0.182. The results are shown in Figure 5.41.

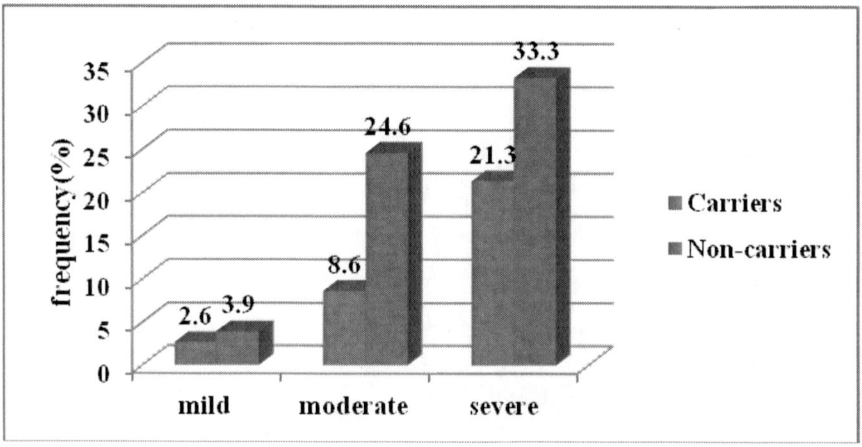

Figure 5.41. Distribution of carriers and non-carrier CFTR mutations with pain.

5.9.3. CFTR Mutations Carrier Status with Diabetes

Analysis of CFTR mutations carrier status with diabetes is presented in the Table 5.21.

Table 5.21. Analysis of CFTR mutations carrier status with diabetes

Tropical Chronic Pancreatitis (n=150)	**Diabetic**	**Non-diabetic**	**OR (95% CI) p-value**
CFTR mutation carriers	30	19	1.743 (0.8701-3.493) 0.1216
Non-carriers	48	53	Reference
Total	78	72	

The CFTR mutation carriers were identified in 20% (30) TCP patients with diabetic and 12.6% (19) of non-diabetic conditions. The non-carriers frequency observed were 32% (48) and 35.3% (53) in diabetic and non-diabetic, respectively, with OR: 1.743, 95%CI: 0.8701-3.493, p- value: 0.121. However, no significant difference was obtained between CFTR mutation and diabetes. The results are shown in Figure 5.42.

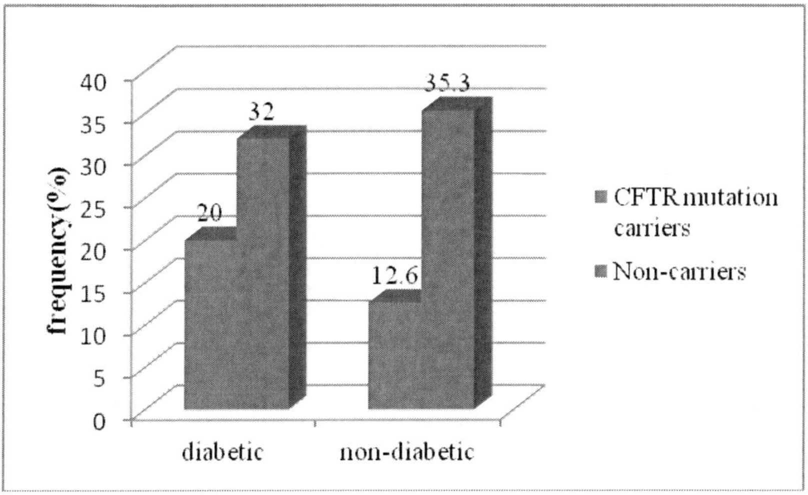

Figure 5.42. Distribution of carriers and non-carrier CFTR mutations with diabetes.

5.9.4. CFTR Mutations Carrier Status with Smoking

Analysis of CFTR mutations carrier status with smoking is presented in the Table 5.22.

Table 5.22. Analysis of CFTR mutations carrier status with smoking

Tropical Chronic Pancreatitis (n=150)	Smoking		OR (95% CI) p-value
	Smoker	Non-smoker	
CFTR mutation carriers	20	29	0.858 (0.429-1.714) 0.726
Non-carriers	45	56	Reference
Total	65	85	

The CFTR mutation carriers were identified in 13.3% (20) TCP patients with smoking and 19.3% (29) of non-smoking nature. The non-carriers frequency of CFTR in smokers was observed to be 30% (45), which was lower as compared to non-smoker TCP patients i.e., 37.3% (56) with OR: 0.858, 95%CI: 0.429-1.714, P-value: 0.726. However, no significant difference was obtained with CFTR mutation and smoking. The results are shown in Figure 5.43.

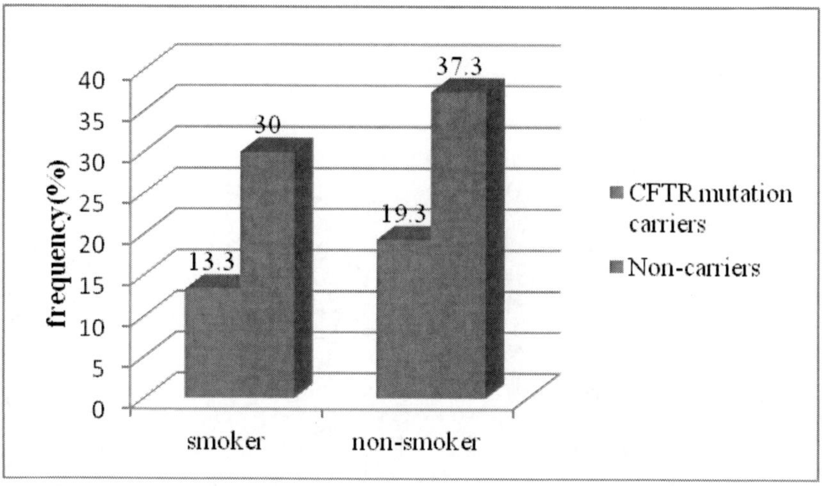

Figure 5.43. Distribution of carriers and non-carrier CFTR mutations with smoking.

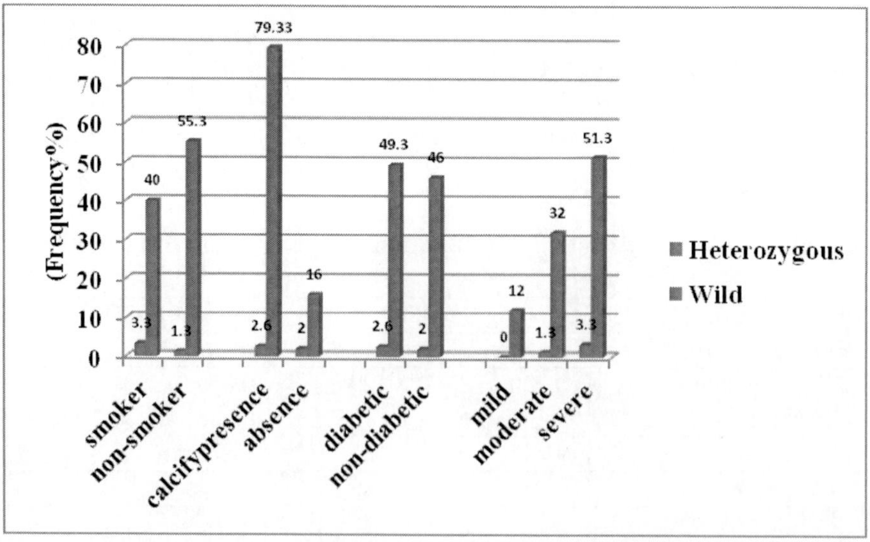

Figure 5.44. Distribution of heterozygous and wild type CTSB (Leu26Val) polymorphism with smoking, calcification, diabetes and pain.

5.10. Genotype-Phenotype Correlation Between CTSB Gene Leu26Val (C76G) Polymorphism and TCP

An endeavour was made to investigate the correlation, if any, between the CTSB gene (Leu26Val) polymorphism with TCP.

Table 5.23. Polymorphism status with phenotype

<table>
<tr><th rowspan="2">Tropical Chronic Pancreatitis (n=150)</th><th colspan="3">Smoking</th><th rowspan="2">OR (95% CI) p-value</th></tr>
<tr><th>Smoker</th><th colspan="2">Non-smoker</th></tr>
<tr><td>Wild</td><td>60</td><td colspan="2">83</td><td>Reference</td></tr>
<tr><td>Heterozygous</td><td>5</td><td colspan="2">2</td><td>3.458 (0.648-18.436)
0.239</td></tr>
<tr><td>Total</td><td>65</td><td colspan="2">85</td><td></td></tr>
<tr><th rowspan="2">Tropical Chronic Pancreatitis (n=150)</th><th colspan="3">Calcification</th><th rowspan="2">OR (95% CI) p-value</th></tr>
<tr><th>Present</th><th colspan="2">Absent</th></tr>
<tr><td>Wild</td><td>119</td><td colspan="2">24</td><td>Reference</td></tr>
<tr><td>Heterozygous</td><td>4</td><td colspan="2">3</td><td>0.268 (0.0564-1.280)
0.110</td></tr>
<tr><td>Total</td><td>123</td><td colspan="2">27</td><td></td></tr>
<tr><th rowspan="2">Tropical Chronic Pancreatitis (n=150)</th><th colspan="3">Diabetes</th><th rowspan="2">OR (95% CI) p-value</th></tr>
<tr><th>Diabetic</th><th colspan="2">Non-diabetic</th></tr>
<tr><td>Wild</td><td>74</td><td colspan="2">69</td><td>Reference</td></tr>
<tr><td>Heterozygous</td><td>4</td><td colspan="2">3</td><td>1.243 (0.268-5.758)
1.00</td></tr>
<tr><td>Total</td><td>78</td><td colspan="2">72</td><td></td></tr>
<tr><th rowspan="2">Tropical Chronic Pancreatitis (n=150)</th><th colspan="3">Pain</th><th rowspan="2">OR (95% CI) p-value</th></tr>
<tr><th>Mild</th><th>Moderate</th><th>Severe</th></tr>
<tr><td>Wild</td><td>18</td><td>48</td><td>77</td><td rowspan="2">1.00</td></tr>
<tr><td>Heterozygous</td><td>0</td><td>2</td><td>5</td></tr>
<tr><td>Total</td><td>18</td><td>50</td><td>82</td><td></td></tr>
</table>

The Leu26Val polymorphism was identified in 3.3% (5) of smokers and 1.3% (2) of non- smokers OR: 3.458; 95%CI 0.648-18.436; P-0.239. Polymorphic status in diabetic and non-diabetic in Heterozygous was 2.6% (4), 2% (3) with (OR: 1.243; 95% CI (0.268-5.758); P-1.00) and in calcification the frequency in heterozygous was 2.6% (4), 2% (3) with OR:

0.268; 95%CI 0.0564-1.280; P-0.110. The results are shown in Table 5.23. No heterozygous polymorphism was found in TCP patients of mild pain. The trend of polymorphic status was similar in all phenotype compared to genotype. No significant association was found between the frequency of the mild-moderate and mild -severe groups, respectively with P-1.0. No association was observed with CTSB and Phenotypes. The results are shown in Figure 5.44.

Table 5.24. MTHFR (C677T) polymorphism with phenotypes

Tropical Chronic Pancreatitis (n=150)	**Smoking**			**OR (95% CI) p-value**
	Smoker	**Non-smoker**		
Wild (CC)	44	46		Reference
Heterozygous(CT)	18	29		0.1881 (0.0749-0.4721) 0.003
Homozygous(TT)	33	10		0.648 (0.3162-1.332) 0.2798
Total	65	85		
Tropical Chronic Pancreatitis (n=150)	**Calcification**			**OR (95% CI) p-value**
	Present	**Absent**		
Wild (CC)	74	16		Reference
Heterozygous (CT)	37	10		0.3083 (0.0356-2.665) 0.427
Homozygous (TT)	12	1		0.800 (0.3307-1.935) 0.6504
Total	123	27		
Tropical Chronic Pancreatitis (n=150)	**Diabetes**			**OR (95% CI) p-value**
	Diabetic	**Non-diabetic**		
Wild (CC)	45	45		Reference
Heterozygous (CT)	25	22		0.710 (0.2023-2.494) 0.755
Homozygous (TT)	8	5		1.136 (0.5606-2.303) 0.8573
Total	78	72		
Tropical Chronic Pancreatitis (n=150)	**Pain**			**OR (95% CI) p-value**
	Mild	**Moderate**	**Severe**	
Wild (CC)	12	33	45	
Heterozygous (CT)	4	17	26	0.001
Homozygous (TT)	2	0	11	
Total	18	50	82	

5.11. GENOTYPE-PHENOTYPE CORRELATION AMONG MTHFR (C677T), ACE I/D GENE POLYMORPHISM AND TROPICAL CHRONIC PANCREATITIS (TCP)

To investigate the genotype-phenotype correlation, of MTHFR (C677T), ACE I/D gene polymorphism with tropical chronic pancreatitis (TCP) and the results are presented in Table 5.24 and Figure 5.45.

The C677T polymorphism was identified in 12% (18) of smokers and 19.3% (29) of non-smokers with OR: 0.1881; 95%CI 0.0749-0.4721; P=0.003. A positive interaction was observed between the 677CT genotype and cigarette smoking with respect to the risk of Chronic Pancreatitis. Significant association was observed with pain P-0.001. No association was found with diabetes and calcification. The results are shown in Figure 5.45.

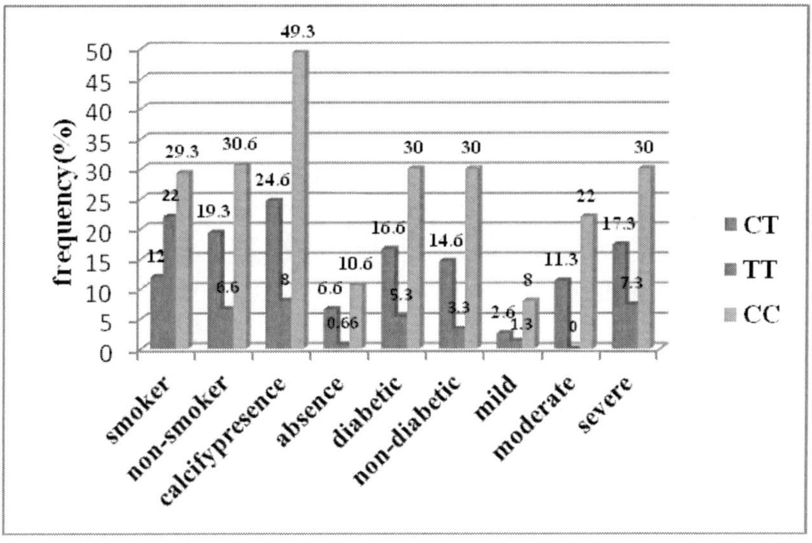

Figure 5.45. Distribution of heterozygous, homozygous and wild type MTHFR (C677T) polymorphism with smoking, calcification, diabetes and pain.

5.12. CORRELATION BETWEEN ACE (I/D) POLYMORPHISM WITH PHENOTYPES

The analysis of the data showing correlation between ACE (I/D) polymorphism with phenotypes is presented in Table 5.25.

The ACE ID polymorphism was not associated with TCP phenotype. The results of frequency distribution of heterozygous, homozygous and wild type and ACE ID polymorphism with phenotype are shown in Figure 5.46.

Table 5.25. ACE (I/D) polymorphism with phenotypes

Tropical Chronic Pancreatitis (n=150)	**Smoking**			**OR (95% CI) p-value**
	Smoker	**Non-smoker**		
Insertion (II)	30	26		Reference
Insertion/Deletion (ID)	20	32		1.846(0.857-3.975) 0.127
Deletion (DD)	15	27		2.077(0.913-4.722) 0.1021
Total	65	85		
Tropical Chronic Pancreatitis (n=150)	**Calcification**			**OR (95% CI) p-value**
	Present	**Absent**		
Insertion(II)	43	13		Reference
Insertion/Deletion (ID)	42	10		0.787(0.3114-1.992) 0.645
Deletion (DD)	38	4		0.348(0.1046-1.159) 0.106
Total	123	27		
	Diabetes			
Tropical Chronic Pancreatitis (n=150)	**Diabetic**	**Non-diabetic**		**OR (95% CI) p-value**
Insertion(II)	30	26		Reference
Insertion/Deletion (ID)	25	27		1.243(0.268-5.758) 1.00
Deletion (DD)	23	19		0.953(0.426-2.128) 1.00
Total	78	72		
Tropical Chronic Pancreatitis (n=150)	**Pain**			**OR (95% CI) p-value**
	Mild	**Moderate**	**Severe**	
Insertion(II)	12	19	25	
Insertion/Deletion (ID)	4	15	33	0.581
Deletion (DD)	2	16	24	
Total	18	50	82	

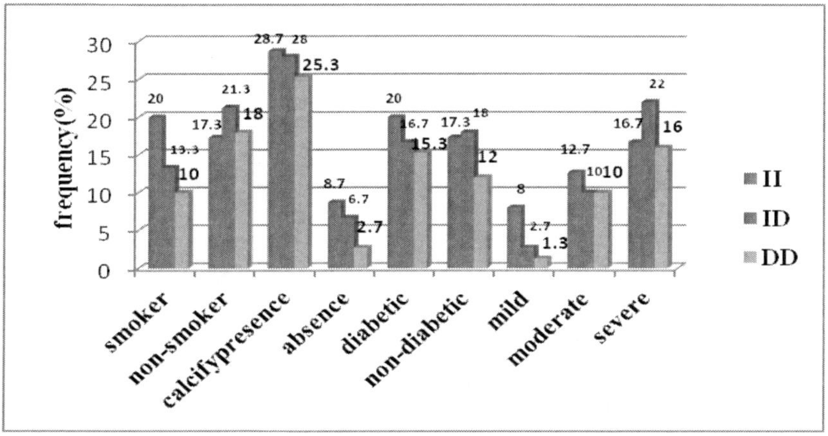

Figure 5.46. Distribution of heterozygous, homozygous and wild type ACEI/D polymorphism with smoking, calcification, diabetes and pain.

5.13. Gene-Gene Interaction

Due to multi-factorial nature of the disease risk we tried to investigate the possible gene-gene interactions. We had taken the genetic mutations of the candidate genes for pancreatitis i.e., SPINK1 CFTR, CTSB, MTHFR and ACE. The results showed that SPINK1 (N34S) alone accounted for the disease causation in 41% of the CP. Only CFTR (ΔF508) gene was mutated in 8.1% of the TCP. Both SPINK1 and CFTR genes were mutated in 50% of TCP group in comparison to 4% of Control group. In association with any of the gene mutations i.e., either SPINK1 (N34S) or CFTR (ΔF508) or both, these factors were able to detect etiology of TCP patients. However, we still did not get any causal factors in 50% of the TCP patients. The analysis of the data is presented in Table 5.26.

Table 5.26. Analysis of the data for gene-gene interactions

Groups	TCP (%) (n=150)	Control (%) (n=150)
SPINK1 mutation	62 (41.3)	03 (2)
CFTR mutation (ΔF508)	13 (8.7)	03 (1.9)
CTSB	07 (4.6)	01 (0.66)
Both genes (SPINK1+CFTR)	75 (50)	06 (4)
SPINK1+CFTR+CTSB	82 (54.6)	07 (4.66)

5.13.1. Combined Effect of SPINK1 and CFTR Gene

We analyzed the SPINK1 polymorphism in association with CFTR genotype in TCP groups. For this we have divided the subject groups in three categories for analysis:

Group A: Neither SPINK1 nor CFTR gene mutations
Group B: Either SPINK1 Polymorphism or presence of CFTR genotype
Group C: Presence of both SPINK1 polymorphism and CFTR genotype

Combination of genotype frequencies and analysis of these three groups are shown in Table 5.27.

Table 5.27. Summary of combination of genotype distribution and analysis

Groups	TCP	Control	P value TCP vs. Control
Group A%	24 (16%)	132(88%)	Reference
Group B%	107 (71.3%)	16 (10.6%)	0.021(0.0115-0.0448)0.227
Group C%	19 (12.6%)	2 (1.3%)	0.001(0.0412-0.08627) 0.18

The distribution of frequency in combination genotype of SPINK1 and CFTR are shown in Figure 5.47.

5.13.2. Combined Effect of SPINK1 and CTSB Gene

Group A: Neither SPINK1 nor CTSB gene mutations
Group B: Either SPINK1 polymorphism or presence of CTSB genotype
Group C: Presence of Both SPINK1 polymorphism and CTSB genotype

Combination genotype frequencies and analysis of three groups are shown in Table 5.28 and Figure 5.47.

The distribution of frequency in combination of genotype of SPINK1 and CTSB are shown in Figure 5.48.

Table 5.28. Summary of Combination genotype distribution and analysis

Groups	TCP	Control	P value TCP vs. Control
Group A%	57 (38%)	144 (96%)	Reference
Group B%	90 (60%)	6 (4%)	0.001(0.0103-0.0607) 0.251
Group C%	3 (2%)	0	0.189(0.0167-2.120) 0.189

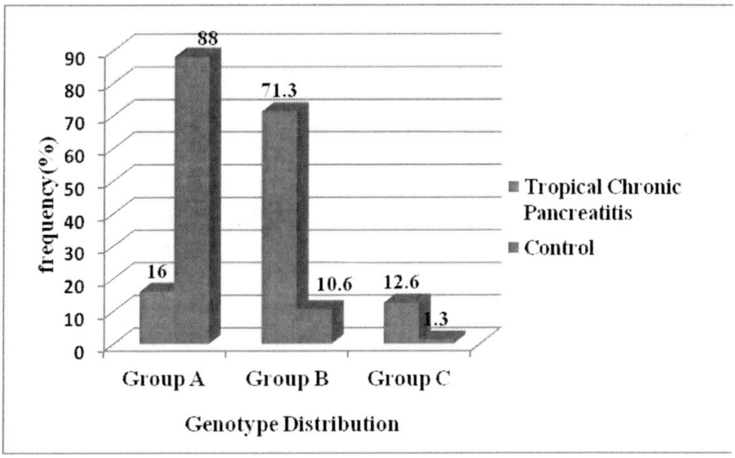

Figure 5.47. Genotype distribution of SPINK1 and CFTR gene.

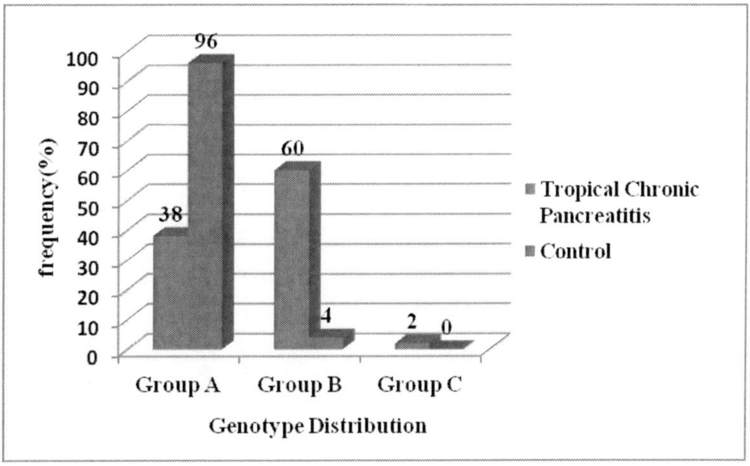

Figure 5.48. Combined distribution of SPINK1 and CTSB gene.

5.14. Extended Family Screening

For extended family screening program, we have followed 10 families, where we have been able to collect the sample of the family members other than proband. Patients were evaluated in families with more than two first- or second-degree relatives by first taking a careful personal and family history. Particular attention is directed to personal risk factors such as cigarette smoking, alcohol use, diabetes, and occupation and for the presence abdominal pain, diarrhea, and abnormal weight loss. We screened for SPINK1 and CFTR gene mutation, as SPINK1 was found in 51% of patients and CFTR in 35% of patients. So we have taken these two important genes for screening. The purpose of the extended family screening was to identify carrier's status of gene mutation among family members and provide genetic counseling to them accordingly. Proband is a term used most often in medical genetics to denote an individual who presents with a disease and whose family is then followed for other investigations.

5.14.1. Proband 1

The proband visited Gastroenterology OPD with a complaint of severe pain in the abdomen and constipation. The proband had a history of alcohol intake of approx 150 ml per week since 20 years of age. Radiography showed heterogeneously enhancing pancreas in region of head, body and tail with multiple hypo dense necrotic areas in pancreatic parenchyma. He had sepsis, which responded slowly to meropenem. He was clinically diagnosed as a case of alcoholic chronic pancreatitis (ACP). Lipid profile values of the proband were as following: Triglyceride=114mg/dl, Total Cholesterol-100mg/dl, HDL Cholesterol= 27mg/dl, LDL Cholesterol= 50mg/dl, VLDL Cholesterol-23mg/dl. Liver function tests showed Serum Aspartate Transaminase-30U/l, Serum Alanine Transaminase-25 U/l, Alkaline Phosphatase -97U/l and Serum Amylase -577IU/L. Pedigree of the family is shown in Figure 5.49.

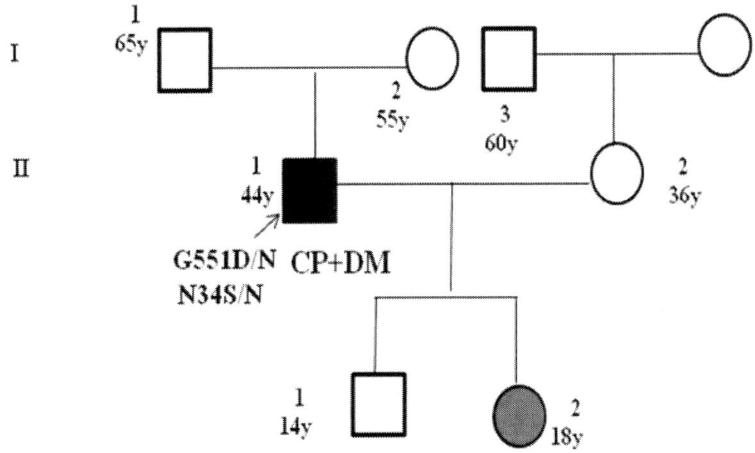

Figure 5.49. Pedigree of family showing family history of Diabetes Mellitus.

The patients were found to be compound heterozygous for SPINK1 gene mutation [N34S] and heterozygous for CFTR gene [G551D/N]. The family study was conducted and found both offspring as trait for Hb E. His daughter also carries G551D mutation in heterozygous state. His brother and his wife both were found normal on haemoglobin variant analysis. There was no family history of pancreatitis.

5.14.2. Proband 2

A case of TCP with atrophied pancreas dilated MPD (minor papillary duct) and coarse calcific foci in MPD was analysed (Figures 5.50 and 5.51). She suffered from recurrent attack of pancreatitis since she was 10 years old. Serum amylase was 98IU/L, which falls in normal range (43-116IU/L) but found increased compared to that normal before the episode around (20IU/L). The patient was found heterozygous for SPINK1 gene mutation [N34S] and heterozygous for CFTR gene [ΔF508/N]. Her brother carried IVS-137T>C mutation in heterozygous state.

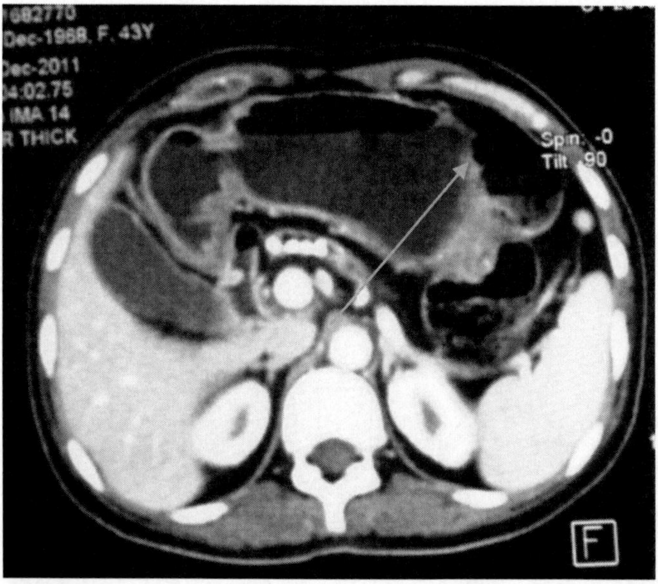

Figure 5.50. Abdominal computed tomography of the patient Atrophy of the pancreatic Parenchyma and numerous calcifications throughout the pancreas.

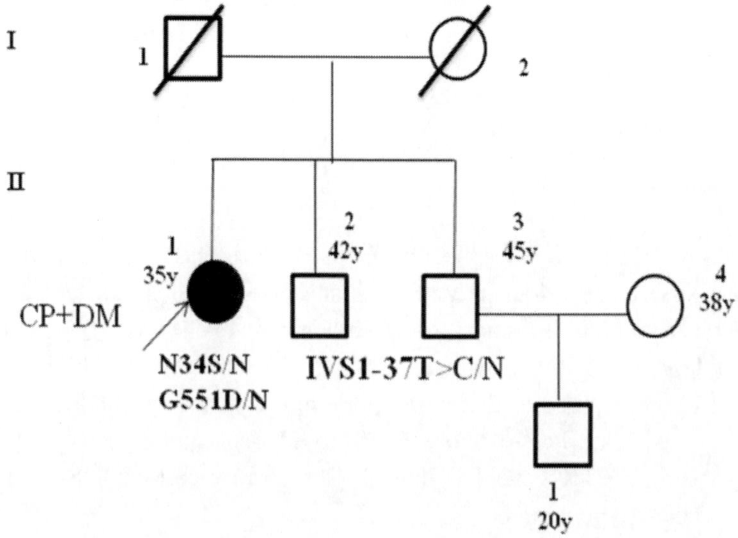

Figure 5.51. Pedigree chart for proband 2.

5.14.3. Proband 3

A 42 year old male had severe six episodes of recurrent pain and weight loss. The age of onset was 35 years. He had no history of alcohol consumption, family history of pancreatitis was not found. Abdominal computed tomography revealed numerous stones in the dilated main pancreatic duct in the pancreas head. He had exocrine insufficiency confirmed by pancreatic function diagnostic test (54.4%; normal range>70%). The proband was found to be heterozygous for SPINK1 [N34S/N] and CFTR gene [G551D/N] mutation. The male offspring of 10 years old was found to possess SPINK1 [N34S/N] polymorphism and CFTR [G551D/N] heterozygous mutation (Figure 5.52).

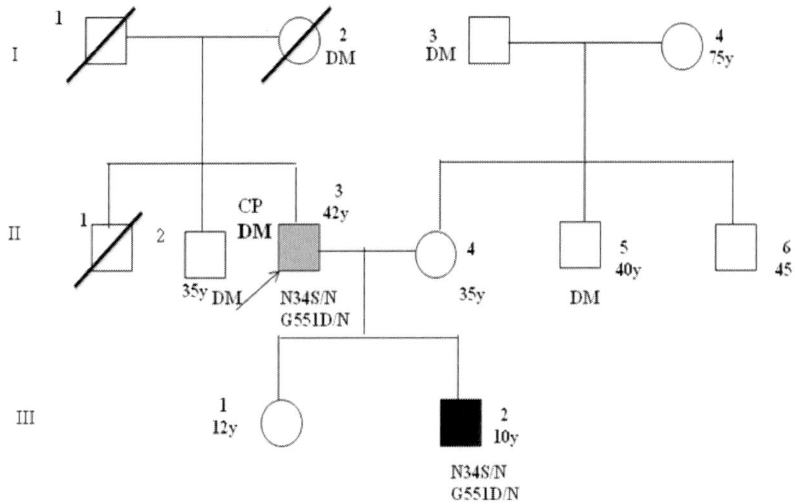

Figure 5.52. Pedigree chart of proband 3.

5.14.4. Proband 4

A 29 year old female patient had recurrent attacks since she was 22 years old with severe weight loss and pain. She was diagnosed with jaundice after onset of pancreatitis. She had Serum Amylase level of 98IU/L belonging to normal range (40-140U/L). Endoscopic Retrograde Cholangiopancreatograpy showed the pancreas divisum from the major papilla demonstrated the main pancreatic duct and the anatomized without depiction of the accessory pancreatic duct depicted in Figure 5.53. Genetic Screening showed this proband with SPINK1 gene polymorphism and CFTR (G551D/N) mutation and the offspring of 8 year old male with CFTR mutation as shown in Figure.5.54.

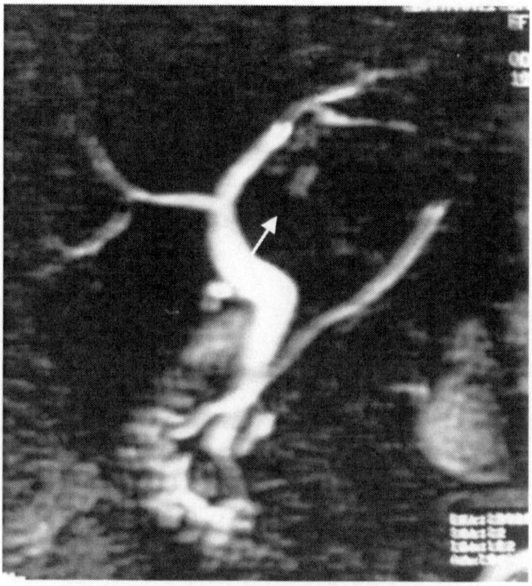

Figure 5.53. MRCP shows the duct of ventral pancreas is not depicted. It shows the enlargement of accessory duct of the pancreas, no connection was observed between the duct.

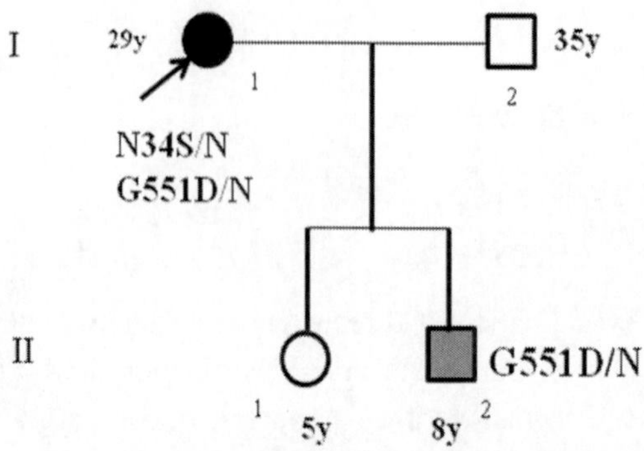

Figure 5.54. Pedigree chart for proband 4.

5.14.5. Proband 5

A 35 year old female patient was found to have no recurrent attacks and pain, but severe weight loss of 10 years with in six month. The age of onset of disease was 29 year. The presentation of diabetes was found in 31 year. Pain was due to congenital anomaly with narrowing of minor papillary duct as shown in Figure 5.55. Genetic Screening showed SPINK1 gene polymorphism and CFTR (R117H/N) mutation in proband and the offspring of 10 years old male with CFTR mutation as shown in Figure 5.56.

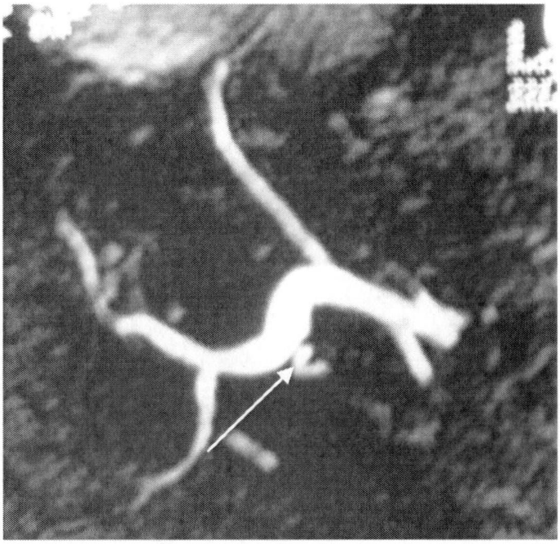

Figure 5.55. MRCP shows that there was no connection betwwen dorsal and ventral duct, depicted of pancreas divisum.

5.14.6. Proband 6

A 40 year old man was referred to our hospital for endoscopic investigation for pain. He suffered from recurrent attacks of pain since he was 27 years old. The diabetes mellitus (DM) was not confirmed in him as he had no prior history of DM. Laboratory data showed an elevation of Serum Amylase 1342IU/L which increased before the elevation or onset of previous attack. Computed Tomography showed the swelling of the pancreas head with scattered tiny calcification. Genetic Screening showed proband with SPINK1 gene polymorphism and his wife had CFTR gene mutation. Offspring of 17 years old male with SPINK1 gene polymorphism and other offspring of 8 years old with CFTR (F508/N) mutation were found. The results are shown in Figure 5.57.

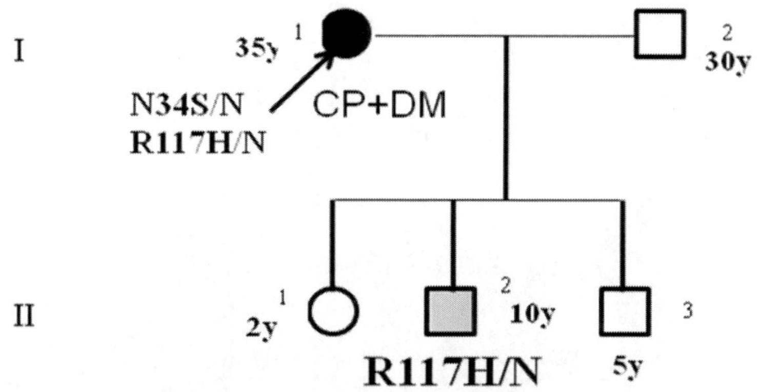

Figure 5.56. Pedigree chart of proband 5.

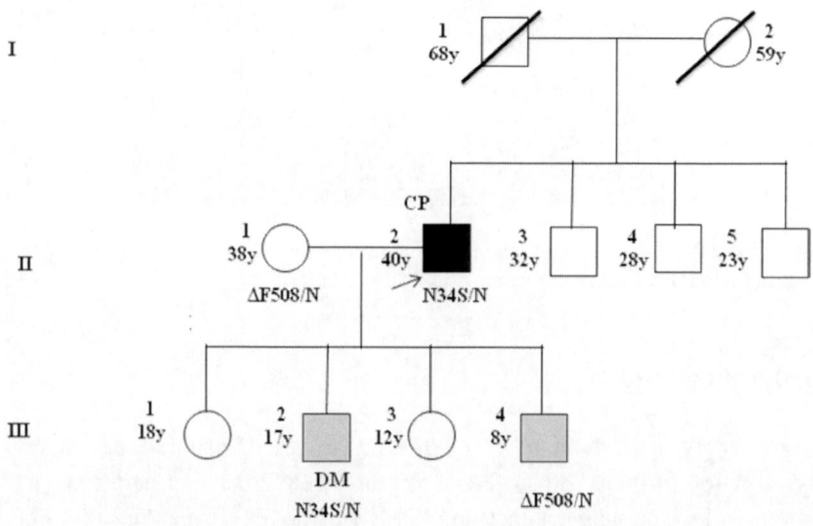

Figure 5.57. Pedigree chart for proband 6.

5.14.7. Proband 7

34 years-old male from Gwalior presented with recurrent episodes of pain and bloating of upper abdomen since 1½ years and pain in the left loin since 1week. The patient had suffered from an attack of acute pancreatitis in January 2008. Thereafter, he had continued to have exacerbations of upper abdominal pain every 2-3 months and was hospitalized elsewhere each time, kept nil orally and treated with IV fluids, antibiotics and analgesics. In between the attacks, he could be on regular pancreatic enzyme preparations and intermittent analgesics. Endoscopic Retrograde Cholangiopancreaticography (ERCP) done on him during August 2008 was normal. A contrast enhanced CT of the abdomen done just prior to admission to our hospital in June 2009 was suggestive of calcification in head region of pancreas with dilated Pancreatic Duct (PD). Serum amylase and lipase levels were higher compared to normal range. A CECT of his abdomen was suggestive of features of chronic calcific pancreatitis. Genetic Screening showed this proband containing SPINK1 gene polymorphism and CFTR (F508/N) mutation and the offspring1 of 11 years old male with CFTR mutation as shown in Figure 5.58.

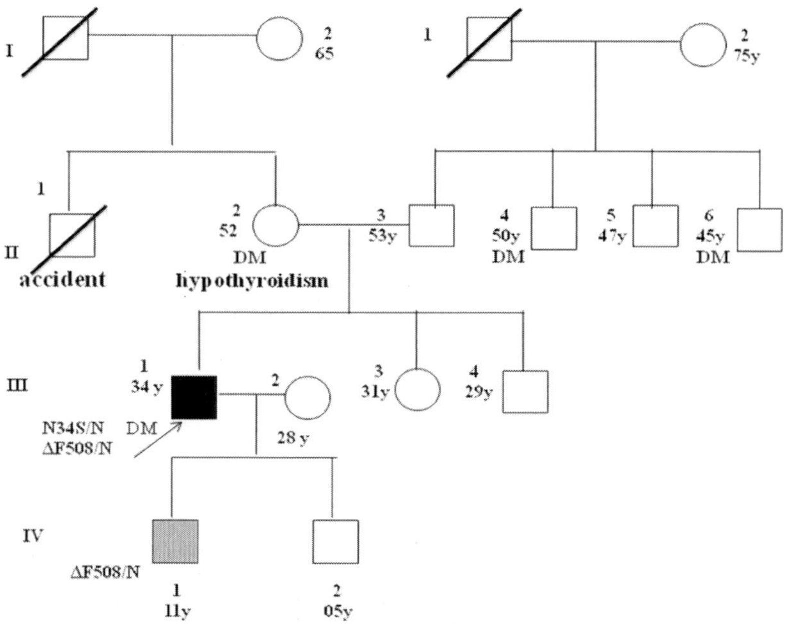

Figure 5.58. Pedigree chart for proband 7.

5.14.8. Proband 8

A 22 years old female was admitted to our hospital with lower abdominal pain and vomiting. The age of onset of disease was 15 years with severe weight loss. The disease progressed with recurrent attack. Laboratory investigations showed the raised levels of Serum Amylase 985IU/L and Lipase 1091. Lipid profile values of proband were as following: Triglyceride = 98mg/dl, Total Cholesterol = 100mg/dl, HDL Cholesterol = 16mg/dl, LDL Cholesterol = 34mg/dl and VLDL Cholesterol-17mg/dl. Liver function tests showed the following values of certain key enzymes: Serum Aspartate Transaminase -25U/l, Serum Alanine Transaminase-19 U/l and Alkaline phosphates - 99U/l. Abdominal Ultrasonography (US) showed a hypo echoic swelling of the entire pancreas as shown in Figures 5.59 and 5.60. In this study, the polymorphisms of SPINK and CFTR gene mutations were not detected. However, it requires further sequencing of SPINK and CFTR genes to identify other novel mutation or possibility of autoimmune pancreatitis.

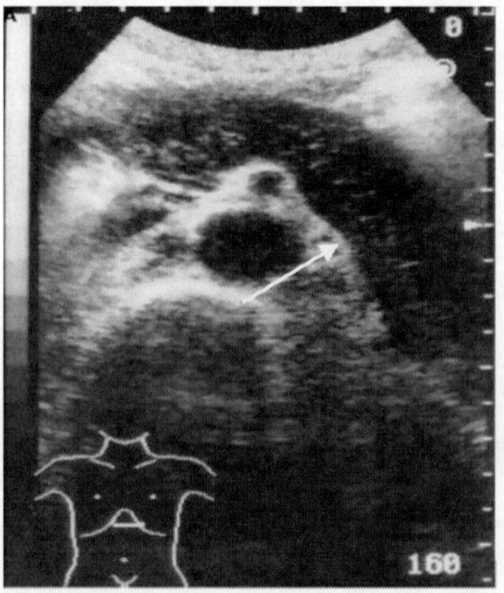

Figure 5.59. Abdominal Ultra sonogram on admission showed diffuse enlargement of the pancreas with hypo echoic images.

5.14.9. Proband 9

A 20 years old male of TCP was admitted to a private nursing home with recurrent fever and pain in abdomen. Recurrent attack appeared since he was six years old. No further disease progression was observed. Ultrasound of abdomen showed chronic calcific pancreatitis with no free fluid, undergone some instrumentation (ERCP). No other symptoms were present. Upon screening, this proband was found to exhibit only SPINK1 polymorphism (IVS3+2T>C/N). N34S/N polymorphism was absent in this proband. CFTR mutation was not found in this proband. IVS3+2T>C polymorphism of SPINK1 gene mutation which causes skipping of exon 3 in SPINK1 gene (Figure 5.61).

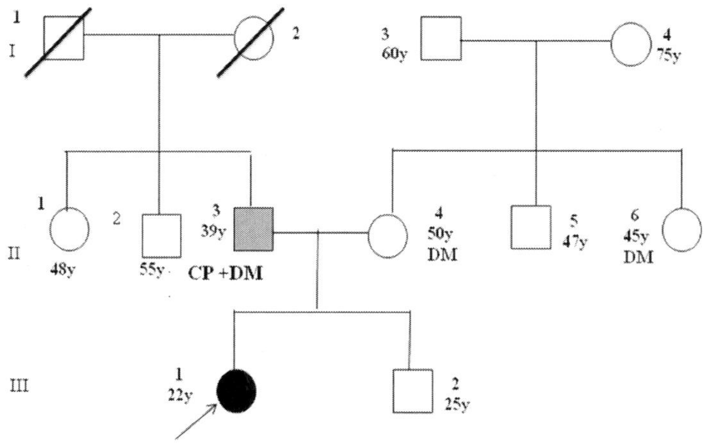

Figure 5.60. Pedigree chart for proband 8.

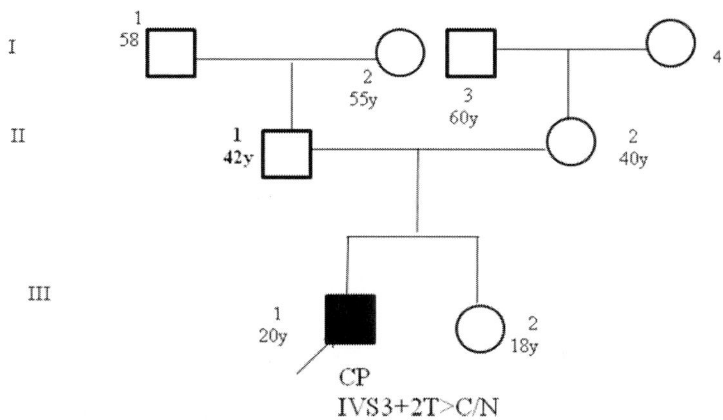

Figure 5.61. Pedigree chart for proband 9.

5.14.10. Proband 10

A 40 year-old man was admitted to the hospital complaining of epigastric pain and high fever. A diagnosis of alcohol-induced CP was made 10 years earlier. Laboratory data on admission showed the following abnormalities: serum amylase: 2909 IU/L (normal range: 42–130IU/L); Prothrombin time: 34% (70–100%); Fibrinogen: <50mg/dl (150–400); DD-dimer: 24.11μg/ml (0.00-1.00μg/ml). Abdominal enhanced computed tomography (CT) revealed presence of a pseudocyst of 2.5cm in diameter at the pancreatic head with upstream dilatation of the PD and fluid collection surrounding the pancreas. Endoscopic retrograde cholangiopancreatography (ERCP) with PD stenting was attempted. Endoscopic treatment can provide short-term relief of abdominal pain in selected patients with CP. On genetic screening proband was found positive for N34S SPINK1 polymorphism. CFTR mutation was not found in this patient as well as in any other members of the proband (Figure 5.62).

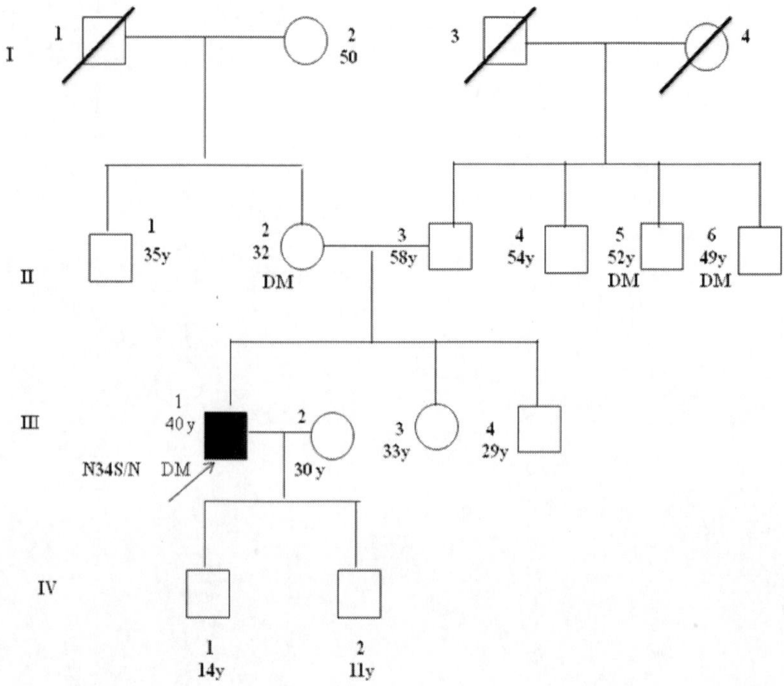

Figure 5.62. Pedigree Chart for proband 10.

Chapter 6

DISCUSSION ON ASSOCIATED MECHANISM: MOLECULAR, GENETIC AND ENVIRONMENTAL ATTRIBUTES TO TROPICAL CHRONIC PANCREATITIS

Tropical Chronic Pancreatitis (TCP) is an incurable, persistent and inflammatory disease characterized by progressive and ultimately irreversible damage to both exocrine and endocrine functions of the pancreas. Genetic and biochemical evidences define a pathological pathway in which a sustained imbalance between intrapancreatic trypsinogen activation and trypsin inactivation result into the development of the disease. Most of the patients included in this study were from low socio-economic strata, possibly because of the location of this tertiary medical care hospital which caters the complicated and untreatable patients referred by medical doctors posted at various Government and private hospitals. The poor quality of lives of majority of patients is associated with inadequate intake of proteins and other nutrients [Duggan et al., 2010]. According to Grant et al. [2011] the factors closely associated with quality, environment, diet and congenital abnormality may augment the threat of the CP disease.

The results from the present study on tropical chronic pancreatitis (TCP) indicate that this disease develops in the first and second decade of life and is seen more commonly in males. Abdominal pain is the most common presenting symptom of TCP. The profile of TCP in the present study seems to be changing with time. Diabetes was found more commonly associated with TCP presentation. The development of pseudocysts is also the most common complication of TCP. One third to half of the patients with TCP had pancreatic calcification but the data obtained on frequency and pattern of calcification in TCP was heterogeneous as some centres reporting higher frequency of pancreatic calcification and ductal calculi whereas some having the pattern and frequency similar to alcohol related TCP [Bhasin et al. 2011]. Diabetes mellitus was significantly more common in calcific pancreatitis group as compared to the non-calcific group. The data from the present study reflect that calcification develops in late stages of TCP associated with advanced endocrine deficiency.

The biochemical profile of controls and TCP patients in the present study indicated increased levels of LDL, TG, VLDL and cholesterol and lower level of HDL. These results are in agreement with those of Diakowska et al. [2005]. They have shown the occurrence of abnormal metabolism of triglycerides fractions in TCP patients of Polish origin.

The clinical features of TCP patients included in the present study indicated pain as a common feature in both the calcific and non-calcific groups. Goulden and his colleagues in 2013 have reported the pathogenesis of pain in TCP patients as a major challenge to physicians, pain specialists, gastroenterologists and surgeons. They reported that upper abdominal pain and back pain with nausea and vomiting could be the main symptoms of TCP. In present study, other environmental factors such as smoking and consumption of alcohol etc increases complications in TCP patients. Similar observations have also been reported by Magno et al. [2010]. They have found that cigarette smoking is a dose-dependent risk factor for acute pancreatitis, recurrent acute pancreatitis and chronic pancreatitis. However, some of chronic alcohol consumers develop recurrent acute pancreatitis but very heavy drinking associates with chronic pancreatitis.

The diabetes related complications in TCP patients have always been posing challenges towards treatment of TCP. The results from the present study have demonstrated that such TCP patients may be prone to ketosis, neuropathy and tuberculosis. No death of such patients was recorded. Similar observations have been reported by other workers in diabetic TCP patients by Barman et al. [2003]; Papita et al. [2012].

6.1. Association of N34S SPINK1 Mutation with Tropical Chronic Pancreatitis

The molecular analysis of TCP patients carried out in present study for the assessment of the types and frequencies of gene polymorphisms into serine protease inhibitor, Kazal type 1 (SPINK1) also known as pancreatic secretory trypsin inhibitor (PSTI). It is a potent anti-protease that is thought to be a major inactivation factor of intrapancreatic trypsin activity. However, trypsin inhibition by SPINK1 is only temporary, because the trypsin-SPINK1-complex itself represents as substrate for trypsin, resulting into a subsequent degradation of the inhibitor molecule and in restoration of the original trypsin activity. Methods of molecular genetics have been used in discovering the pathogenesis of TCP. Some studies have ascribed involvement, controversial though, of the NS34 mutation of SPINK1 gene which occurs with varied frequencies in particular populations of patients and plays differential role in the etiology of various forms of chronic pancreatitis [Matsubayashi et al. 2003; Shimosegawa et al. 2006; Garg et al. 2009].

N34S is a missense mutation in which a A→G transition at nucleotide101 in exon3, results in Asparagines to Serine substitution at amino acid 34. N34S is the most common mutation identified with respect to tropical chronic pancreatitis in various populations. In this study, N34S (heterozygous) mutation in 62 (41.3%) cases and 3 (2%) in controls was recorded which shows significant association of N34S with TCP risk (OR: 19.4, 95%CI: 1.06-356.05, p-value: 0.006). N34S heterozygous mutation was more prevalent in comparison to homozygous mutation. There was no phenotypic correlation was found in relation to homozygous or heterozygous mutation. Thus, it seems that N34S SPINK1 mutation is not disease inducer rather it is disease modifier mutation. These results were in agreement with those reported by Matsubayashi et al., 2003.

In 2002, four different research groups investigated Indian and Bangladeshi patients suffering from TCP, and all reported a strong association with the SPINK1 N34S alteration [Chandak et al.2002, Hassan et al.2002, Bhatia et al.2002, Schneider et. al.2002]. Altogether, 351 patients and 973 control subjects were investigated in these studies. Approximately 9% of patients were homozygous for N34S and 29% heterozygous, compared to 0.2% and 4.3% in control individuals. Chandak et al. 2002 observed in 3 out of 68 (4.4%), but in none of 100 control subjects, a G>T transversion in the SPINK1 promoter region at position −215 relative to the ATG initiation codon (c.1–215G>T) was found. Interestingly, N34S is also very common in Indian subjects suffering from alcohol-related chronic pancreatitis. Ten out of 41 (24.4%) affected individuals carried at least one N34S mutated allele [Chandak et al. 2004]. A more comprehensive study in Bangladesh with 37 TCP patients confirmed the high proportion of N34S mutations in FCDP patients (55%) and TCP (20%). On balance it is clear that the association of N34S is the most evident for CP compared to other CP subtypes with an allele frequency from 8.8 to 41.6 percent [Aoung et al. 2008].

In another study by Midha et al. [2010] in Idiopathic CP patients, SPINK1 N34S mutation was present in 42% of patients with idiopathic CP (vs. 4% controls, p<0.001) and 17% of patients with alcoholic CP (p=0.016 compared with controls). The results of the present study in Indian subjects have indicated the frequency of 42% in CP showed similar trend of frequency and strong genetic susceptibility due to SPINK1 mutation. In one such study, 18 out of 96 unrelated paediatric patients, a c.101A>G transition leading to substitution of asparagines by serine at codon 34 (p.N34S) was found. This variant was present in only 1 out of 279 control subjects (OR 62.2, P<1 10–10). Six patients were homozygous for this mutation [Witt et al. 2000]. A relatively low frequency of SPINK1 mutations is seen in ACP patients. A comprehensive study in 274 ACP patients demonstrated that 5.8% of ACP patients were SPINK1 carrier's compared to only 0.8% in controls [Witt et al. 2001]. These findings were confirmed by reports from other workers [Thread Gold et al.2002, Drenth et al. 2002].

The findings concerning the NS34 of SPINK1 gene mutation and ACP relationship in the Polish population are in contrast with *Gąsiorowska* who found no correlations between the NS34 of SPINK1 gene mutation and ACP in the group of adult Poles. However, their study was focused on the relationship to idiopathic pancreatitis (p< 0.05) and they investigated a smaller group of patients (34 with alcoholic pancreatitis and 14 with idiopathic pancreatitis) [Gąsiorowska et al. 2011]. The results from the present study revealed that SPINK1 gene might act as a genetic predisposing factor for CP irrespective of the etiology. In contrast, Peláez-Luna et al. [2005] have reported that there was an association between SPINK-1 N34S mutation and CP, but linkage studies have failed to show linkage between the disease and the SPINK-1 locus.

Modeling and familial clustering suggests that SPINK-1 mutations modify the disease by lowering the threshold for its development from other genetic or environmental factors, but by themselves do not cause disease [Peláez-Luna et al. 2005]. In Finnish population, the studies conducted by Lempinen et al.

2005 have shown that the SPINK1 N34S mutation was significantly associated with an increased risk of CP. The association of the N34S mutation with alcoholic CP was marginally stronger than in earlier studies, whereas in the Finnish population in general, this mutation was significantly more frequent than reported elsewhere. However, in Romanian population, the N34S mutation was found to be a weak risk factor for alcoholic CP [Diaconu et al. 2009].

6.2. Association of IVS3+2T>C Mutation with Tropical Chronic Pancreatitis

SPINK1 provides the first line of defense against prematurely activated trypsinogen by physically blocking the active site of trypsin. The IVS3+2T>C (c.194+2T>C) mutation is a loss of functional splicing mutation; it affects the consensus splicing donor site in intron 3 and may cause skipping of the entire exon 3, where the trypsin-binding site is located [Ota et al., 2010]. The phenotypic variability of the homozygous IVS3+2T>C mutation in SPINK1 gene in CP patients has been established by this group. However, the results of the present study indicated IVS3+2T>C (heterozygous) mutation in 10 (6.7%) CP cases and 1 (0.67%) in controls which shows significant association of IVS3+2T>C mutation with TCP risk. A sole report of mutated SPINK1 in a CP patient outside the Indian subcontinent exists [Snabbon et al. 2006]. Recently, a Thai group published a case report of a patient with fibrocalculous pancreatic diabetes (FCPD) and a heterozygous SPINK1 variant, c.194+2T>C (IVS3+2T>C), which represents the second most common pathogenic SPINK1 variant in white Caucasians.

Chandak and colleagues have concluded that the c1.-215G>T and c.1–215G>A variants may lie in an unknown cis-acting element and thereby affect transcription of mutated SPINK1 with an already compromised functional capacity. Reddy and Prasad in 2011 have indicated that two common haplotypes, c.101A>G (p.N34S) and c.-215G>A, and four intronic alterations of SPINK1 gene may increase the risk for CP in the Asia Pacific region. However, the c.1–215G>A alteration is in contrast to c.1–215G>T, in complete linkage disequilibrium with another SPINK1 variant, c.194+2T>C [Kaneko et al. 2001, Kume et al. 2005, Kume et al. 2006]. This transition affects splice donor site at position 2 of intron 3, which is highly conserved in eukaryotes [Witt et al. 2000]. The Analysis of the mutated mRNA showed a truncated SPINK1 due to skipping of exon 3 [Kume et al. 2006]. Thus, the pathogenic significance of the c.1–215 variants remains uncertain. The IVS3 + 2T >C mutation affects the splicing donor site that is highly conserved in eukaryotes [Buratti et al. 2004].

6.3. Association of IVS1-37T>C Mutation with Tropical Chronic Pancreatitis

The results of the present study revealed the occurrence of IVS1-37T>C (heterozygous) mutation in 11 (7.3%) cases and 1 (0.67%) in controls which showed significant association with CP risk. Thread gold et al. 2002 have shown that N34S; IVS1–37T 1 C mutation was associated with familial, idiopathic and autoimmune CP. Three of 8 (38%) patients with familial pancreatitis had the N34S mutation, in agreement with the previous report showing a strong association between N34S mutation and familial pancreatitis. N34S; IVS1–37T 1 C mutation in 4 of 31 patients with idiopathic CP. Thus, 7 of 39 (18%) patients with familial or idiopathic CP carried this mutation. This frequency was compatible with the original report by Witt et al. [2000] showing the high incidence (19%) of N34S mutation in patients with idiopathic CP.

Another study by Japanese showing the association of N34S mutation and CP [Truninger et al. 2002; Kuwata et al. 2001] have reported that 3 of 24 (13%) Japanese patients with familial pancreatitis, and 1 of 15 (7%) patients with juvenile pancreatitis carried the N34S mutation. Thus, one explanation for the high N34S frequency in this study may result from careful selection of CP patients with well-defined cases. N34S mutation was found with sequence variants (IVS1-37 T>C). The results of the present study indicated that one of these variants was in the compound heterozygous state which ruled out gross deletions or insertions of any part of the coding or intronic sequence of SPINK1. Another study by Macarena et al. in 38 Italian subjects of idiopathic chronic pancreatitis, IVS1-37 T>C polymorphism was found in 3 subjects and it was found in linkage with N34S polymorphism.

6.4. ASSOCIATION OF ΔF508 MUTATION WITH TROPICAL CHRONIC PANCREATITIS

In the present investigation, the subjects when screened for the seven variants (mutations: ΔF508, G542X, G551D, R117H, W1282X and S549N, polymorphism: IVS8-5T) to find out the association of CFTR gene mutation and polymorphism with severity of TCP, significantly higher frequency of CFTR gene variants among TCP cases (25.39%) was observed as compared to the controls (7.92%). Of the five variants screened, ΔF508 mutation (OR: 4.65, 95%CI: 1.29-16.674, p-value: 0.020) and IVS8-5T variant (OR: 2.2, 95% CI: 0.66–6.74, p-value: 0.004) were found to be associated with TCP. There are not many reports available to suggest the association of these mutations in TCP cases. However, some existing western reports indicate the association of these mutations in CFTR gene with cystic fibrosis [Hughes et al. 2001] and lung cancer [Peadar et al. 2000].

The ΔF508 is the most common mutation identified in the CFTR gene, with a reported frequency of 66% worldwide as compared to 19-44% in Indian patients with cystic fibrosis (CF) responsible for 70% of abnormal CF gene [Prasad et al. 2010]. In ΔF508 mutation, there is three-base-pair deletion that produces an in frame deletion of a phenylalanine (F) at position 508 (NBD1 domain). Most of the studies in India and other populations have been done with respect to CF and congenital bilateral absence of vas deferens (CBAVD) [Prasad et al. 2010]. One study tested 134 patients with CP, including 60 cases with idiopathic and 71 cases with alcohol-induced disease, for 22 CFTR mutations [Sharer et. al.1998]. Eighteen patients (13.4%), including 12 with ICP (20%), were heterozygous for a CFTR mutation. The frequency of CFTR mutations in alcohol-related CP was twice, and in ICP four times higher, than expected. In the other study, 17 CFTR mutations in 27 patients with idiopathic CP were investigated [Cohn et al. 1998]. Seven patients (25.9%) had at least one CFTR mutation and 1 patient was compound heterozygous. The frequency of CFTR mutations in idiopathic CP was six times higher than expected. Both studies, however, investigated the most common CFTR mutations only. Sharer and Cohn [1998] showed the link between cystic fibrosis and CP conditions which indicated abnormal sweat chloride contents as well as pancreatic ductal obstruction due to inspissated secretions. Moreover, some the CF patients suffer from recurrent attacks of pancreatitis. In the present study, higher frequency of delF508 (heterozygous) mutation among CP cases 13 (8.7%) was recorded as compared to controls 3 (1.9%). The analysis of allele frequency of

CP cases and controls in present investigation indicated significant different in mutant allele frequency of CP cases than the controls where as wild allele frequency remains same in both these groups. The data establishes significant associations of heterozygous genotypes and mutant allele frequency with CP patients.

In Serbian population significant association of ΔF508 mutation was observed with CP (p=0.032) [Nikolić et al. 2011]. Midha et al. [2010] in a case- control study observed strong genetic susceptibility of ΔF508 mutation with TCP [Midha et al. 2010]. In another such study, a significant association of ΔF508 mutation was observed with TCP, the value of frequency being 11.8% [Bhatia et al. 2000]. The results from present investigation were in agreement with the previous studies from west which showed that CFTR mutation frequency is higher in idiopathic pancreatitis than alcoholic pancreatitis [Perri et al. 2003].

The ΔF508 mutation belongs to class II CFTR mutation. Class II mutations are characterized by defect in processing or trafficking of the CFTR protein in the endoplasmic reticulum. CFTR mutation may result in the ductal obstruction due to abnormal secretion of bicarbonate rich fluid which may account for pancreatitis [Riordan et al. 1989].

Unlike these studies, very recently Awasthi et al. [2012] have shown heterozygous ΔF508 mutation in 4 (1.6%) Asthma cases and 3 (1.2%) controls indicating no significant association between ΔF508 mutation and asthma (OR: 1.3, 95%CI: 0.296-6.046, p-value: 0.70). In contrast, Lee demonstrated that the groups of CFTR gene mutation carriers (Korean population) had significant association with CP cases. Their results also revealed that interactions between multiple genetic variants in cis affected the final function of the gene products p=0.032 [Lee et al. 2003].

6.5. Association of G542X Mutation with Chronic Pancreatitis

G542X, a nonsense mutation (class I) with G→T transition at nucleotide 1756 (exon 11) undergoes in the mutation of the codon (GGA) for the amino acid glycine at 542 to the translational stop codon TGA. G542X is the second most common CFTR mutations identified in various populations with reference to CF [Ahmed et al. 2003]. The results of the present study indicated the higher frequency of G542X (heterozygous) mutation among TCP cases 10

(6.7%) as compared to controls 3(2%) (OR: 3.5, 95%CI: 0.94-12.986, p-value: 0.085). The mutant allele frequency in TCP cases was also greatly different from the controls. However, no association either of the above two factors was observed with CP. In a report presented by Reboul et al. [2003] the presence of the S1235R mutation--in trans with regard to G542X—has been speculated to be responsible for the idiopathic chronic pancreatitis (ICP) phenotype.

6.6. Association of G551D Mutation with Tropical Chronic Pancreatitis

G551D is a missense mutation (class III) in which a G→A transition at the nucleotide1784 located in exon11 takes place in many CF cases [Michael et al. 2012]. It results into Glycine to Aspartic acid substitution at amino acid 551. G551D is the third most common CFTR mutation identified with respect to CF in various populations. G551D has been identified and reported in Indian population (n=100) in one individual with CF [Sharma et al. 2009b]. The results of the present study demonstrated the presence of heterozygous G551D mutation in 9 (6%) cases and 4 (2.7%) controls. The data showed no association of G551D with TCP risk (OR: 2.3, 95%CI: 0.70-7.74, p-value: 0.25). We could not come across any such study reporting the association of G551D mutation with TCP.

6.7. Association of R117H Mutation with Tropical Chronic Pancreatitis

The R117H mutation of exon IV of the CF gene is a G→A substitution at position 482. One of the mutations in the extended mutation analysis is R117H, which is considered to be a mild CF mutation associated with a broad phenotype, ranging from no clinical disease to CF with suppurative lung disease [Balnaves et al. 1995]. As per recommendation of Balvanes et al if R117H is detected, 5T testing is recommended. If both are found, then additional testing for haplotyping should be performed to determine whether they are located on the same chromosome or not [Strom et al. 2002]. The results of the present study have demonstrated R117H (heterozygous) mutation in 2 (1.3%) TCP cases and 1(0.7%) controls, which shows no association of R117H with TCP risk. One such study has reported the mutation

ΔF508/R117H mutation with CP [Sharer et al. 1998]. Ravnik Glavac et al. [2000] have presented an evidence that hereditary pancreatitis is genetically heterogeneous disorder. Though they have initially found a single mutation R117H in the cationic trypsinogen gene followed by a second mutation, N21L, in all affected members of five unrelated hereditary pancreatic families, their association with the disease could not get confirmed.

6.8. Association of S549N Mutation with Tropical Chronic Pancreatitis

S549N is a missense mutation in which a G→A transition at nucleotide 1778 in exon11 results in Serine to Asparagine (S→N) substitution at amino acid position 549. It is one of the common CFTR gene mutations identified in the Indian population with reference to CF [Shastri et al. 2008; Sharma et al. 2009]. The results of the present study showed the frequency of heterozygous S549N mutation among TCP cases to be 2.0% (3) as compared to the controls 0.66 % (1). However, it was not found statistically significant in terms of its association with TCP risk.

6.9. Association of IVS8-5T Polymorphism with Tropical Chronic Pancreatitis

Three length variants of a polypyrimidine tract within the splice acceptor site in intron 8 of the CFTR gene have been found to be associated with varying degrees of exon 9 splicing as detected mainly in the CF cases [Kiesewetter et al. 1993; Ooi et al. 2012]. One of their copies of the CFTR gene has a problem with mRNA splicing. This splicing problem results from an abnormally short polythymidine tract (5T) in intron 8 of the gene. Three variants occur at this splicing site, termed 5T, 7T, and 9T, depending on the number of thymidines. The 5T variant occurs on 5% of chromosomes in the general population, and differs from the 7T and 9T variants because it hinders splicing of CFTR mRNA. In individuals with the 5T variant, many copies of their CFTR mRNA are missing an essential exon (e.g., exon 9). Thus, the 5T allele (at this site in intron 8) causes CBAVD by partially reducing the level of functional CFTR (without exon 9, CFTR cannot function). Patients with one AF508 allele and one 5T allele (AF508/5T) do not develop CF because they produce enough properly spliced and functional CFTR to prevent lung disease, but they do not produce enough functional CFTR to protect the vas deferens [Kiesewetter et al. 1993].

One common mutation of the CFTR gene has been implicated in the pathogenesis of TCP, the 5T variant of the variable length polythymidine tract in intron8 (IVS8). The CFTR gene contains a sequence of 5, 7 or 9 polythymidine bases (poly T sequence) located at the splice acceptor site of intron8. The 5T variant sequence decreases the efficiency of intron8 splicing and is considered a mild mutation. The most frequent genotype was 9T/9T genotype in all the two groups. The 5T/9T (P=0.15; OR=3.4; 95%CI= (0.63-1.9) and 7T/9T (P=0.1; OR=1.6 95%CI (0.776-3.45) genotypes were associated with the increased risk to tropical chronic pancreatitis in comparison to healthy control though the P values were not significant [Midha et al. 2010] in Idiopathic chronic pancreatitis patients showed that the CFTR gene, present in nine patients with idiopathic CP had mutations and 41 patients had polymorphisms (50% vs 10% controls, p<0.001). Only a single study investigated the prevalence of CFTR mutations in TCP patients and only 2/18 patients carried a mutant allele [Bhatia et al. 2000].

Initial studies on the role of CFTR mutations and the 5T allele in ACP patients refused a correlation [Malats et al. 2001; Haber et al. 2001]. Subsequent studies, however, did detect an association (10-18%) between CFTR and ACP. All of the CFTR mutations seem to have a role in ACP but the results are controversial. [Monaghan et al. 2000; Truninger et al. 2001]. Earlier to these reports, couple of studies had shown a correlation between CFTR mutations and ICP [Sharer et al. 1998; Cohn et al. 1998]. They reported 10/27I CP patients carried a CFTR mutation and/or the so-called 5T allele. The 5T allele reduces the expression of functional CFTR and is associated with patients with CBAVD. In the same year another case study investigated 134 CP patients: 71 patients with ACP, 60 patients with ICP and 3 with metabolic CP. Eighteen patients, of which 12were ICP patients, had a mutation [Sharer et al. 1998]. In another study by Maltas et al. (2001) 5T allele was found 5.5%.5T allele carriers with cancer consumed significantly less alcohol than non-carriers (p-0.038).

6.10. Association of CTSB Gene Leu26Val Variants with Severity of Tropical Chronic Pancreatitis

Cathepsin B is an enzymatic protein belonging to the peptidase (or protease) families. In humans, it is encoded by the CTSB gene. The protein encoded by this gene is a lysosomal cysteine protease composed of a dimer of disulfide-linked heavy and light chains, both produced from a single protein precursor. It is a member of the peptidase C1 family [Saluja et al. 1987]. It is presumed to perform an essential role in intracellular activation of trypsinogen. However, most of the circumstantial evidences are based on its *in vitro* capability to activate trypsinogen and its co-localization in secretary granules containing digestive enzymes [Watanabe et al. 1984; Figarella et al. 1988]. The results of the present study indicated Leu26Val (heterozygous) mutation in 4.6% (7) TCP cases and 0.66% (1) in controls. These results reflected no association of Leu26Val with CP risk. Mahurkar and co-workers in 2006 performed a mutational analysis of CTSB and found an association between CP and a c.76C>G transversion in exon 3, leading to leucine by valine exchange at codon 26 (p.L26V). Investigating 306 Indian patients with TCP and 330 controls, the 26V allele was significantly overrepresented in patients (minor allele frequency 0.46) compared to control subjects allele frequency of 0.29 and P value was P-0.013[Mahurkar et al. 2006]

6.11. Association of MTHFR Gene Variants C677T with Severity of Tropical Chronic Pancreatitis

The MTHFR gene contains a 2.0-kbp coding region with 11 exons and is located on chromosome 1p 36.3. It is a key enzyme in folate metabolism that catalyzes the conversion of 5, 10-methylenetetrahydrofolate (5, 10-methylene THF) to 5-methyltetrahydrofolate (5-methyl THF) a predominant circulatory form of folate and methyl donor for the remethylation of homocysteine to methionine [Fodinger et al. 2000]. The results of the present study have shown a significant association between the MTHFR C677T polymorphism and risk of CP in Indian population. Individuals carrying the homozygous TT variant genotype conferring low enzyme activity had a 2 fold increased risk of developing TCP compared to the individuals with the CC wild-type or the heterozygous CT genotype. The results of one such study published so far by

Ivan and Jelena in [2008] have indicated increased frequency (51%) of the C677T polymorphism in chronic pancreatitis patients in Serbian population; the data however, was not found statistically significant with (P-0.458) [Ivan et al. 2008].

The allele frequency in Europeans was 24%–40% (34), 26%–37% in Japanese (18) and >11% in the African American population. [Papapetrou et al.1996; Stevenson et al. 1999; Ulvik et al. 2001]. The results obtained from the present study indicated 32.6% genotype prevalence of C677T polymorphism and it was found to be statistically significant. The data indicated that the MTHFR 677TT genotype had a significant effect on the risk of CP. The complex interactions of these genetic and environmental factors in CP may play an important role in disease progression. Such knowledge may have important implications for the primary management of TCP [Singh et al. 2013].

6.12. Association of ACE Gene Polymorphism with Severity of Tropical Chronic Pancreatitis

The systemic hormonal renin-angiotensin system (RAS) has important physiological functions in the regulation of blood pressure, fluid and electrolyte balance. They are mainly executed by angiotensin II, the product of hydrolysis of angiotensin I by angiotensin-converting enzyme (ACE). In the pancreas, major components of such a local pancreatic RAS have been implicated in the regulation of acinar digestive enzyme secretion, islet hormonal secretion and ductal anion secretion [Leung et al. 2003]. The data obtained from the present study demonstrated ACE ID to be in 50 (33.3%) CP cases and 47 (31.3%) in controls, which showed no association of ACEI/D with TCP risk. Several studies conducted in past have demonstrated that ACE inhibitors and angiotensin II type 1 receptor blockers prevent pancreatic stellate cell activation and fibrosis [Kuno et al. 2003]. Another such study investigated the ACE I/D variant in 171 Indian subjects with TCP and compared the genotype and allele frequencies with 99 ethnically matched healthy controls [Bhaskar et al. 2006]. No significant differences with TCP per se, as well as with fibrosis or progression of the disease, were observed by Bhaskar et al. [2006]. Our results are concordance of Bhaskar et al. results.

6.13. Genotype and Phenotype Correlation

Genotypic and phenotypic correlations among the mutations in the key genes in TCP cases and certain phenotypic characteristics have also been evaluated in the present study. This study could establish a correlation between SPINK1 gene polymorphism and TCP. The present results indicated that SPINK1 N34S polymorphism was identified in 32% cases with calcification, 42% cases with mild to moderate pain, 39% cases with diabetes and 34% cases with smoking habits. The analysis of results indicated a significant correlation of this mutation with calcification and diabetes in TCP patients whereas no association with pain and smoking could be established. The results of this study regarding evaluation of genotypic and phenotypic correlation between CFTR gene mutation and TCP revealed that CFTR mutation carriers were identified in 26.6% patients with calcification, 15.6% cases with mild to moderate pain, 20 % with diabetes and 13.3% with smokers; displaying a significant correlation of CFTR mutation between calcification and TCP without any correlation between TCP and pain or diabetes or smoking. The analysis of results using the data obtained for evaluation of genotype-phenotype correlation between CTSB gene (Leu26Val) polymorphism and TCP suggested that Leu26Val polymorphism carriers were not having any significant correlation between TCP cases and the diabetes, smokers or mild to moderate pain. However, the data obtained on assessment of a correlation among the MTHFR (C677T) and ACE ID gene polymorphism and TCP indicated that there was significant increase in the number of insertion, insertion/deletion and deletion mutations in the smokers than non smokers. However, in diabetic's insertion and deletion mutations were more dominant than normal subjects. All of these mutations were dominant in TCP cases with severe pain followed by those with moderate and mild pains.

6.14. Extended Family Screening

The pattern of probands during extended family screening of 10 randomly selected TCP cases revealed presence of some common characteristics e.g. all of the probands suffered from pain for many years in one or the other areas of their stomach. The abdominal pain in all these TCP cases was associated with weight loss. Excluding a few, all of them displayed increase in the activities of key marker enzymes such as transaminases, amylase and lipase. The mutation in SPINK1 gene was observed to be a very common characteristic in TCP cases screened so far, though the mutations varied at different codons. In contrast, the pattern of mutations in the CFTR gene was not uniform in all these probands screened; some of the TCP cases did not show presence of mutations in this gene. All the tested probands displayed heterogeneous enlargement of pancreas; some of them showing a sign of calcification as well. Only two probands were tested for the levels of cholesterol and different lipoproteins. The results demonstrated increase in the level of total cholesterol and HDL. Out of 10 probands screened, only one was alcoholic and the other was diabetic in nature. A survey of published literature, however, does not indicate any such reports on the screening of characteristics of probands and their offspring's suffering from TCP.

Chapter 7

SUMMARY OF STUDY ON TROPICAL CHRONIC PANCREATITIS AND CONCLUSION

The present three years study included 150 cases of chronic pancreatitis (TCP) and 150 age and sex matched controls collected from October 2009 to March 2013. Maximum numbers of patient were recruited in the months of April and May. Mean age of patients was 49.9 ± 14.8 years. Of which 105 (56.6%) were males. Maximum numbers of patients were in the age group of 20 to 40 years. The age of presentation of disease occurs in Ist decade. Among 150 cases of CP, 49% of TCP patients were recruited with no other clinical complications. 42% of TCP was with Diabetes Mellitus with exocrine, endocrine insufficiency. 8% of Pancreas Divisum (PD) was registered. Though PD itself is not a cause of pancreatitis but 8% of TCP with Pancreas Divisum (PD) and 1% of TCP with pancreas divisum plus diabetes mellitus were registered in this study.

The geographical distribution of TCP patients was also a reflection of the patho-physiology of the disease. 8% of the patients were from Basti and 7% from Gorakhpur. The results showed that there was common denominator of the region, which reflects the poor standard of nutrition. Moreover, the climate of this region is favourable in progression of disease. Large segments of population in this region use insufficient amount of protein in their diet. So the factors closely associated with quality, environment, diet and congenital abnormality increase the threat of the disease. As the number of patients recruited was less, so it does not show the overall frequency.

The number of individuals having classical risk factors viz diabetes; smoking and family history were found to be significantly higher in patients group. The TCP patients (150) and controls (150) were further classified into three groups: Group I consisted of diabetics/non diabetics, group II contained smokers/Nonsmokers and group III consisted of family history/no family history of TCP. The ratio of diabetics/non-diabetics was 42:49 in TCP as compared to 28:72 in control groups. The percentage of smokers in TCP group was 39% more than the control group.

An insignificant difference in the ratio of male: female was noted in both the TCP patients and control groups. The 105 males and 45 females were included in the TCP patients group, whereas 104 healthy males and 46 healthy females were included in the control group of this study. A significant (p=0.001) difference for mean values of BMI and weight were noted between TCP patients and controls.

A complete lipid profile like (triglycerides, total cholesterol, HDL cholesterol, LDL cholesterol and VLDL cholesterol in control and patients indicated that the levels of very low density lipoprotein (VLDL) and low density lipoprotein (LDL) were significantly higher in TCP patients than in controls with significant association. However, the level of high density lipoprotein (HDL) was lower in TCP patients group. A higher % of smokers and diabetes were observed in patients group (p<0.001) compared to controls.

The male to female ratio in TCP patients was 2.3:1.0. The mean age of diagnosis was found to be 50.8±16.7 years. The presentation of the disease was 30.5 years in the calcific group and 23 years in the non-calcific group. Pain was the commonest presenting symptom and it was present in 65% of patients. The age of onset of diabetes mellitus was 36.2±11.27 years. The duration of pain in calcific and non calcific groups was 2.19 years. In addition, 39% of the patients were smokers. Pancreas divisum was found in 8% and calcification was observed in 54% of patients. Steatorrhea was observed in 4.3% and coleolithiasis in 16.5% of cases. The history of all the patients indicate though the age of onset of the disease 26.04±9.8 is quiet early but confound diagnosis was usually established at later stages 35.8±16.7 years Cigarettes smoking was found quiet common in 39% of cases and diabetes get precipitated in second and third decade of life in TCP patients, that leads to complications and that leads to complications in duration of calcification and pain. Neuropathy and tuberculosis were present in 1% and 2% of patients.

The heterozygous (101A>G) polymorphism was identified 41.3% in TCP cases and 2% in controls. Mutant allele frequency of N34S was 24% in TCP cases as compared 1% in controls. A significant difference between the genotype and allele frequency was observed between the two groups (p<.005).

The heterozygous IVS3+2T>C polymorphism was identified 6.7% in TCP cases and 0.67% in controls. Mutant allele frequency of IVS3+2T>C was 3.3%

in cases as compared 0.3% in controls. Higher proportion of polymorphism among TCP cases was observed as compared to controls. A significant difference between the genotype and allele frequency was observed between the two groups (p<0.005).

The heterozygous IVS1-37T>C polymorphism was identified 7.3% in TCP cases and 0.66% in controls. Mutant allele frequency of IVS1-37T>C was 3.7% in TCP cases as compared to 0.33% in controls (p-value: 0.008). We observed higher proportion of polymorphism among TCP cases as compared to controls. A significant difference between the genotype and allele frequency was observed between the two groups (p<0.05).

The heterozygous ΔF508 mutation was identified 13 (8.7%) in TCP cases and 3(1.9%) in controls. Mutant allele frequency of ΔF508 was 4.3% in cases as compared 1% in controls. We observed higher proportion of ΔF508 mutation among cases as compared to controls. A significant difference between the genotype and allele frequency was observed between the two groups (p<0.05).

The heterozygous G542X mutation was identified 10 (6.7%) in TCP cases and 3 (2%) in controls. Among TCP group the mutant allele frequency of G542X was found 3.3% as compared to 1% in controls. The proportion of G542X mutation was higher among cases as compared to controls. However, no significant difference between the genotype and allele frequency was observed between the case and control group (p<0.05).

The (heterozygous) G551D mutation was identified 9 (6%) in TCP cases and 4 (2.7%) in controls. The proportion of G551D mutation was significantly higher among cases as compared with controls. The mutant allele frequency of G551D was found 3% in cases as compared to 1.3% in controls. After comparing the allele frequencies between the two groups it was observed that a mutant allele frequency was significantly higher among TCP as compared to controls. However, no significant difference between the genotype and allele frequency was observed between the CP and control group (p<0.05).

The heterozygous R117H mutation was identified 2 (1.3%) in TCP cases and 1 (0.77%) controls. The proportion of G551D mutation was significantly higher among TCP as compared to controls. The mutant allele frequency of G551D was found 0.66% in CP as compared to 0.33% in controls. However, no significant difference between the genotype and allele frequency was observed between the TCP and control group (p<0.05).

The heterozygous S549N mutation was identified in 3 (2.0%) cases and 1 (0.6%) controls. Among case group the mutant allele frequency of S549N was 1.0% as compared to 0.3% in controls. The higher proportion of S549N mutation was observed among cases as compared to controls. However, no significant difference between the genotype and allele frequency was observed between the two groups ($p<0.05$).

One common mutation of the CFTR gene has been implicated in the pathogenesis of chronic pancreatitis, the 5T variant of the variable length polythymidine tract in intron8 (IVS8). The CFTR gene contains a sequence of 5, 7 or 9 polythymidine bases (poly T sequence) located at the splice acceptor site of intron8. The 5T variant sequence decreases the efficiency of intron8 splicing and is considered a mild mutation. The most frequent genotype was 9T/9T genotype in all the two groups. The 5T/9T and 7T/9T genotypes were associated with the increased risk to chronic pancreatitis in comparison to healthy control though the P values were not significant. This shows a trend of variant poly T sequence to be associated with the disease. The variant Poly T sequence i.e. 5T allele was present in 8.6% of TCP patients as compared to 1% in control, and exhibited a trend for increased for increased risk to tropical chronic pancreatitis patients.

The heterozygous C76G polymorphism was identified 7 (4.6%) in TCP cases and 1 (0.66%) in controls. Among TCP cases group the mutant allele frequency of Leu26Val was found 2.3% as compared to 0.3% in controls. The frequency was found higher in TCP cases as compared to control. However, no significant difference between the genotype and allele frequency was observed between the two groups.

The ACE (ID) mutation was identified 50 (33.3%) in CP cases and 47 (31.3) in controls, among TCP case group, I allele frequency of was 55.3% as compared to 53% in controls and D allele frequency was (45%) in cases as compared to (47%) in control. However, no significant difference between the genotype and allele frequency was observed between the two groups.

The heterozygous C677T polymorphism was identified 49 (32.6%) in CP cases and 12 (8%) in controls. Among CP case group the mutant allele frequency of C677T was found 26.3% as compared to 6% in controls. The higher proportion of C677T polymorphism was observed among cases as compared to controls. A significant difference between the genotype and allele frequency was observed between the two groups.

In order to achieve secondary objective, mutants of SPINK1 gene variants among cases were compared with wild type. Mutants were defined as those subjects which were found heterozygous for any of the three variants (polymorphism: N34S, IVS3+2T>C, and IVS1-37T>C) studied whereas; Wild type are those subjects which were homozygous for the wild type allele. Analysis of N34S carrier frequency after categorizing our study cohort in to groups by age showed interesting results. The < 20 yrs groups had a carrier frequency of 41.5 % (22 of 53) which is significantly higher than that of 36% (35 of 97) in the 20-60 years old group (p<0.016). We categorized the study cohort according to etiology and then compared the SPINK1 N34S positive and negative patients in each category as a function of various phenotypic markers.

The SPINK1N34S polymorphism was identified in 48 (32%) cases with calcification and in 18(12%) of mutated patient calcification was not found. Calcification as factor associated with N34S mutation showed similar trends suggested that mutation status directly related to the calcification. However, a significant difference between the polymorphism positive and polymorphism negative was observed between the two groups.

The SPINK1N34S polymorphism was identified in 12 (8%) cases with mild intermittent pain with 30 (20%) had moderate constant pain as compared with SPINK1 N34S polymorphism negative 18(12%) of mild and 25(16.6%) had moderate pain, respectively, with no significant association of patients with mild to moderate pain with N34S mutation, it might another factor predominant in disease progression. When compared the mutated SPINK1 N34S mutation in patients with mild pain and compared to severe constant pain we found frequency 46 (30.6%) with no significant association between two groups with p-value 0.811.

Diabetes mellitus as a feature of pancreatic endocrine insufficiency was prevalent in 39 (26%) of chronic pancreatitis patients with diabetes as predisposing factors with mutated SPINK1N34S polymorphism as compared to 27(18%) of non-diabetic patients. A comparison of SPINK1 polymorphism frequency in TCP patients with diabetes and without diabetes show the trend of disease severity suggesting that mutation status is directly related to the presentation of diabetes. Negative SPINK1 N34S polymorphism in diabetes was found 27(18%) as compared to non-diabetic 57(38%). Comparing two parameters we found significant association and three times the risk of disease.

Prevalence of N34S SPINK1 mutation 34(22.6%) in patients with smoker was similar in patients with non-smoker 32(21.3%). However, no association was observed between N34S polymorphism and smoking. This may be due to other factors associated with other TCP groups as the prevalence of N34S mutation was comparable in both the groups. The negative N34S mutation prevalence in smoker 20.6% as compared to nonsmoker 35.3%, this showed variability in the mutation status with different groups.

The categorization of various phenotypic features in patients with and without SPINK1 mutations carriers vs. non-carriers was comparable. It is now considered that SPINK1 gene mutation play a modifier role in function of various phenotypic features.

In 150 TCP patients carrier's frequency of SPINK1 mutations was 88 (58.6%) compared to non-carriers frequency 62(41.3%). Prevalence of mutations was higher in more than 50% of patients and was found to be strongly associated with chronic pancreatitis but the variability was observed in mutation status, 44% of N34S mutation was observed in TCP patients as compared to other 14% of mutation of SPINK1 alone a contributing factor. Biochemical investigations like lipid profile (triglycerides, total cholesterol, HDL cholesterol, LDL cholesterol and VLDL cholesterol). The value of serum high-density lipoprotein (HDL) cholesterol is significant (p-0.002) as it showed comparably same values in lower range with lower values of HDL in carriers groups as compared to non-carriers. However the levels of serum triglyceride, total cholesterol, low-density lipoprotein (LDL) cholesterol and very low-density lipoprotein (VLDL) no significant association between two groups. Significant association was observed in Serum Lipase (p-0.012) as values were almost same between carriers and non-carriers group.

The categorization of various phenotypic features in patients with and without SPINK1 polymorphism carriers vs. non-carriers was comparable. It is now considered that SPINK1 gene polymorphism play a modifier role in function of various phenotypic features. In 150 TCP patients carrier's frequency of SPINK1 polymorphism was 88 (58.6%) compared to non-carriers frequency 62(41.3%). Prevalence of mutations was higher in more than 50% of patients and was found to be strongly associated with chronic pancreatitis but the variability was observed in mutation status, 44% of N34S polymorphism was observed in TCP patients as compared to other 14% of mutation of SPINK1 alone a contributing factor. Biochemical investigations like lipid profile (triglycerides, total cholesterol, HDL cholesterol, LDL cholesterol and VLDL cholesterol). The value of serum high-density lipoprotein (HDL) cholesterol is significant (p-0.002) as it showed comparably same values in lower range with lower values of HDL in carriers groups as compared to non-carriers. However the levels of serum triglyceride, total cholesterol, low-density lipoprotein (LDL) cholesterol and very low-density lipoprotein (VLDL) were found no significantly association between two groups. Significant association was observed in Serum Lipase (p-0.012) as values were almost same between carriers and non-carriers group.

The carrier SPINK1 polymorphism was identified in 57(38%) of TCP patients have calcification and 20(13.3%) with absence of calcification. The most similar trend was observed in non-carriers with calcification and frequency was 51(34%) (OR: 0.590, 95%CI: 0.602-2.510, p-value: 1.229). However, no significant difference between the frequencies was observed between the two groups.

The carrier SPINK1 polymorphism was identified in 5(3%), 15(10%) and 42(28%) of patients with mild, moderate and severe pain, respectively. No association was observed when compared mild and severe. The trend of mutation frequency was same with non-carriers SPINK1 mutation in severe pain 40(26.6%) with no significant association was observed with (p-0.026). The results are shown in Figure 8.3.2. So the presentation and age of onset of pain with different decades had no association with SPINK1 polymorphism, there may be another factors associated with the type of pain which might mask the effect of other factors.

The frequency of carriers SPINK1 polymorphism in diabetic patients was 33(22%) compared to 29(19.3%) of non-diabetic. Non-carrier frequency was 45(30%) and 43(28.6%), respectively, in diabetic and non-diabetic patients with no association (OR: 1.041, 95%CI: 0.763-1.419, p- value: 0.868). The results were shown in Figure 8.3.3. The exact relationship between the diabetes and TCP is not clear, although there is an overlap between the phenotypes and SPINK1 polymorphism carrier frequency.

The carrier frequency of SPINK1 polymorphism in smoker and non-smoker were 34(22.6%) and 32(21.3%), respectively. Non-carrier frequency were 31(20.6%) and 53(35.3%) in both the groups. We found no association between the groups with carriers frequency (OR: 0.574, 95%CI: 0.298-1.109, p- value: 0.135).

The CFTR mutation carriers was identified in 40(26.6%) patients of calcification and 10(6.6%) with absence of calcification. The non-carriers frequency of CFTR in calcification was observed 60(40%) as compared to patients with absence of calcification 40(26.6%) (OR: 2.6, 95%CI: 1.198-5.937, p-value: 0.016). However, significant ($p<0.05$) difference between the frequency was observed between the two groups.

The CFTR mutation carriers were identified in 4(2.6%) TCP patients with mild pain, 13(8.6%) moderate and 32(21.3%) of severe pain. Non-carriers frequency observed were 14(9.3%), 37(24.6%) and 50(33.3) in mild, moderate and severe pain, respectively. No significant association was observed between frequencies of mutation between the two group's mild, moderate and mild, severe, respectively, P-value 0.182.

The CFTR mutation carriers were identified in 30 (20%) TCP patients with diabetic and 19 (12.6%) with non-diabetic conditions. The non-carriers frequency observed were 48 (32%) and 53 (35.3%) in diabetic and non-diabetic, respectively, (OR: 1.743, 95%CI: 0.8701-3.493, p- value: 0.121). However, no significant difference between the frequencies was observed between the two groups.

The CFTR mutation carriers were identified in 20(13.3%) TCP patients with smoking and 29 (19.3%) with non-smoking behaviour. The non-carriers frequency of CFTR in smokers was observed to be 45(30%), which was lower as compared to non-smoker TCP patients i.e. 56(37.3%) (OR: 0.858, 95%CI: 0.429-1.714, p- value: 0.726). However, no significant ($p>0.05$) difference in the frequency was observed between the two groups.

The Leu26Val polymorphism carriers were identified in 5(3.3%) of smokers and 2(1.3%) of non-smokers (OR: 3.458; 95%CI 0.648-18.436; P-0.239). Polymorphic status in diabetic and non-diabetic in Heterozygous was 4(2.6%), 3(2%) with (OR: 1.243; 95% CI (0.268-5.758); P-1.00) and in calcification the frequency in heterozygous was 4(2.6%), 3(2%) with (OR: 0.268; 95%CI 0.0564-1.280; P-0.110). No heterozygous polymorphism was found in TCP patients of mild pain. The trend of polymorphic status was similar in all phenotype compared to genotype. No significant association was found between the frequency of the mild-moderate and mild-severe groups, respectively, with P-1.00). No association was observed in CTSB with Phenotypes.

Due to multi-factorial nature of the disease risk, the possible gene-gene interactions were investigated. We had taken the genetic mutations of the candidate genes for pancreatitis i.e. SPINK1 CFTR, CTSB, MTHFR and ACE. The results showed that SPINK1 (N34S) alone accounted for the disease causation in 41% of the TCP. Only CFTR (ΔF508) gene was mutated in 8.1% of the TCP. Both SPINK1 and CFTR genes were mutated in 50% of TCP group in comparison to 4% of HC group. In association with any of the gene mutations i.e. either SPINK1 (N34S) or CFTR (ΔF508) or both, these factors were able to detect etiology of TCP patients. However, we still did not get any causal factors in 50% of the TCP patients.

Family screening was done in subjects found positive (carriers) for CFTR, SPINK1and CTSB gene mutations defined as probands. There were 10 Families (with effected proband) for extended family screening. Of these, 10 families visited us and agreed to give blood sample. The purpose of the extended family screening was to identify more carriers of gene mutation among family members and give genetic counseling to the family of the probands.

The pattern of probands during extended family screening of 10 randomly selected TCP cases revealed presence of some common characteristics e.g. all of the probands suffered from pain

for many years in one or the other areas of their stomach. The abdominal pain in all these TCP cases was associated with weight loss. Excluding a few, all of them displayed increase in the activities of key marker enzymes (transaminases, amylase and lipase). The mutation in SPINK1 gene was observed to be a very common characteristic in TCP cases screened so far, though the mutations varied at different codons. In contrast, the pattern of mutations in the CFTR gene was not uniform in all these probands screened; some of the TCP cases did not show presence of mutations in this gene. All the tested probands displayed heterogeneous enlargement of pancreas; some of them showing a sign of calcification as well. Out of 10 probands screened, only one was alcoholic and the other was diabetic in nature.

The proband 1 was found compound heterozygous for SPINK1 gene mutation [N34S and IVS3+2(T-C)] and heterozygous for CFTR gene [G551D/N]. Proband 2 was found heterozygous for SPINK1 gene mutation [N34S] and heterozygous for CFTR gene [ΔF508/N]. His brother carries IVS-137T>C mutation in heterozygous state. Proband 3 was found heterozygous for SPINK1 gene mutation [N34S] and heterozygous for CFTR gene [G551D/N]. Offspring was found [G551D/N] heterozygous but no mutation was found in SPINK1gene. Proband 4 was with SPINK1 gene polymorphism and CFTR (G551D/N) mutation and the offspring of 8 year old male with CFTR mutation. Proband 5 was with SPINK1 gene polymorphism and CFTR (R117H/N) mutation and the offspring of 10 years old male with CFTR mutation. Proband 6, showed SPINK1 gene polymorphism and his wife had CFTR gene mutation. Proband 7 contained SPINK1 gene polymorphism and CFTR (F508/N) mutation and the offspring of 11 years old male with CFTR mutation. In Proband 8, polymorphisms of SPINK and CFTR gene mutations were not detected. Proband 9, exhibited only SPINK1 polymorphism (IVS3+2T>C/N). IVS3+2T>C polymorphism was found to cause skipping of exon 3. Proband 10, was observed to contain SPINK1 polymorphism. CFTR mutation was not found in this patient as well as in any other members of the proband.

An important goal of research on TCP is to understand the genetic and environmental triggers for pancreatitis and the factors that lead to variations in its natural history. The screening of SPINK1, *CFTR* gene, family screening in *CFTR* mutation carriers and study on expression analysis will undoubtedly help in understanding the role and molecular mechanism of SPINK1 and

CFTR gene in tropical chronic pancreatitis and better characterization gene mutation in Indian population. Therefore, further studies among different populations with pancreatitis and well-defined clinical data will help to verify these preliminary results and attempt to characterize a possible influence of gene mutation in etiology of a tropical chronic pancreatitis.

Recently, some other genes were identified as pancreas specific and play a role in pancreatitis. So a thorough investigation of these genes such as CTRC, CASR, Cathepsin D, keratin 8 may give us a better understanding of this complex disease.

References and Citations

Adler DG, Lichtenstein D, Baron TH, et al. The role of endoscopy in patients with chronic pancreatitis. *Gastrointestinal Endoscopy.* 2006; 63:933–937.

Ahmad SA, Wray C, Rilo HL, Choe KA, Gelrud A, Howington JA,. Chronic pancreatitis: recent advances and ongoing challenges. *Current Problems Surgery* 2006;43:127-238.

Alberti KGMM, Zimmet PZ. Definition, diagnosis and classification of diabetes mellitus and its complications: I. Diagnosis and classification of diabetes mellitus: provisional report of a WHO consultation. *Diabetes Medical* 1998; 78: 539-53.

Aoun E, Chang CC, Greer JB, Papachristou GI, Barmada MM, Whitcomb DC. Pathways to injury in chronic pancreatitis: decoding the role of the high-risk SPINK1 N34S haplotype using meta-analysis. *PLOS ONE* 2008; 3: e2003.

Apte MV, Pirola RC, and Wilson JS. Molecular mechanisms of alcoholic pancreatitis. *Digestive Diseases.* 2005; 23: 232–240.

Audrézet MP, Chen JM, Le Maréchal C, Ruszniewski P, Robaszkiewicz M, Raguenes O. Determination of the relative contribution of three genes-the cystic fibrosis transmembrane conductance regulator gene, the cationic trypsinogen gene, and the pancreatic secretary trypsin inhibitor gene-to the etiology of idiopathic chronic pancreatitis. *European Journal of Human Genetics* 2002; 10:100–6.

Augustine P, Ramesh H. Is tropical pancreatitis premalignant? *American Journal of Gastroenterology* 1992; 87:1005-8.

Awasthi S, Maurya N, Agarwal S, Dixit P, Muthuswamy S, Singh S. Association of CFTR gene mutation with bronchial asthma and its severity in Indian children: A case-control study. *Annals of Human Biology*. 2012; 39: 113–121.

Axon AT, Classen M, Cotton PB, Cremer M, Freeny PC, Lees WR. Pancreatography in chronic pancreatitis: international definitions. *Gut.* 1984; 25(10):1107-12.

Balaghi, M., Horne, D., Woodward, S. and Wagner, C., Pancreatic one-carbon metabolism in early folate deficiency in rats. *American Journal of Clinical Nutrition.* 1993; 58:198–203.

Balaji LN, Tandon RK, Tandon BN, Banks A. Prevalence and clinical feature of chronic pancreatitis in southern India. *International Journal of Pancreatology.*1994; 15:29-34.

Balnaves ME, Bonacquisto L, Francis I,. The impact of newborn screening on cystic fibrosis testing in Victoria, Australia. *Journal of Medical Genetics* 1995; 32:537–42.

Ulmasov Barbara, Zekuan Xu, Talkad Vanita, Oshima Kiyoko, Brent A. Tetri Neuschwander. Angiotensin II signaling through the AT1a and AT1b receptors does not have a role in the development of cerulein-induced chronic pancreatitis in the mouse. *American Journal of Physiology*.2010.

Barman KK, Premalatha G, Mohan V. Tropical chronic pancreatitis. *Postgraduate Med J* 2003; 79:606–615.

Barman KK, Premalatha G, Mohan V. Tropical chronic pancreatitis. *Postgraduate Med J* 2003; 79: 606-615.

Bhasin DK, Rana SS, Chandail VS, Singh G, Gupta R, Kang M, Sinha SK, Singh K. Clinical profile of calcific and non-calcific chronic pancreatitis in north India. *J Clinical Gastroenterology;* 2011;45:546-50.

Bhaskar S, Reddy DN, Mahurkar S, Rao GV, Singh L, Chandak GR. Lack of significant association of an insertion/deletion polymorphism in the angiotensin converting enzyme (ACE) gene with tropical calcific pancreatitis. *BMC Gastroenterology.*2006;6:42.

Bhatia E, Choudhuri G, Sikora SS, Landt O, Kage A, Becker M. Tropical calcific pancreatitis: strong association with SPINK1 trypsin inhibitor mutations. *Gastroenterology.* 2002; 123:1020–5.

Bhatia E, Durie P, Zielenski J, Lam D, Sikora SS, Choudhuri G, Tsui LC. Mutations in the cystic fibrosis transmembrane regulator gene in patients with tropical calcific pancreatitis. *American Journal of Gastroenterology.* 2000; 95:3658-3659.

Bolan PJ, Fink AS. Endoscopic retrograde cholangiopancreatography in chronic pancreatitis. *World J Surg.* 2003; 27:1183-91.

Boulling A, Maréchal C, Trouvé P, Raguénès O, Chen JM, Férec C. Functional analysis of pancreatitis-associated missense mutations in the pancreatic secretary trypsin inhibitor (SPINK1) gene. *European J Human Genetics.* 2007; 15:936–42.

Bozkurt T, Braun U, Leferink S, Gilly G, Lux G. Comparison of pancreatic morphology and exocrine functional impairment in patients with chronic pancreatitis. *Gut.*1994; 35:1132-6.

Buratti E, Baralle M, De Conti L, Baralle D, Romano M, Ayala YM, Baralle FE. HnRNP H binding at the 5′ splice site correlates with the pathological effect of two intronic mutations in the NF-1 and TSHβ genes. *Nucleic Acids Research.* 2004; 32: 4224–4236.

Casals T, Aparisi L, Martinez-Costa C, Giménez J, Ramos MD, Mora J, Diaz J, Boadas J, Estivill X, Farré A. Different CFTR mutational spectrum in alcoholic and idiopathic chronic pancreatitis. *Pancreas.* 2004; 28:374-379.

Chandak GR, Idris MM, Reddy DN, Bhaskar S, Sriram PV, Singh L. Mutations in the pancreatic secretory trypsin inhibitor gene (PSTI/SPINK1) rather than the cationic trypsinogen gene (PRSS1) are significantly associated with tropical calcific pancreatitis. *Journal of Medical Genetics.* 2002; 39:347–51.

Chandak GR, Idris MM, Reddy DN, Mani KR, Bhaskar S, Rao GV. Absence of PRSS1 mutations and association of SPINK1 trypsin inhibitor mutations in hereditary and nonhereditary chronic pancreatitis. *Gut.* 2004; 53:723–8.

Chari ST, Mohan V, Pitchumoni CS, Viswanathan M, Madanagopalan N, Lowenfels AB. Risk of pancreatic carcinoma in tropical calcifying pancreatitis: an epidemiologic study. *Pancreas.1994*; 9:62-66.

Chari ST, Mohan V, Jayanthi V, Snehalatha C, Malathi S, Viswanathan M, Madanagopalan N. Comparative study of the clinical profile of alcoholic pancreatitis and tropical chronic pancreatitis in South India. *Pancreas* 1991; 7:2–58.

Chase CW, Barker DE, Russell WL, Burns RP. Serum amylase and lipase in the evaluation of acute abdominal pain. *American Surgery* 1996; 62:1028-33.

Cohn JA. Reduced CFTR function and the pathobiology of idiopathic pancreatitis. *J Clinical Gastroenterology.*2005; 39:70-77.

Cohn JA, Kenneth MD, Friedman BA, Noone PG, Relation between mutations of the cystic fibrosis gene and idiopathic pancreatitis. *New England Journal of Medicine* 1998, 339:653-658.

Comfort MW, Steinberg AG. Pedigree of a family with hereditary chronic relapsing pancreatitis. *Gastroenterology*. 1952; 21:54-63.

Copenhagen Pancreatic Study Group. An interim report from a prospective epidemiological multicentre study. *Scand Journal of Gastroenterology*.1981; 16:305-12.

Curry CA, Eng J, Horton KM. CT of primary cystic pancreatic neoplasm: can CT be used for patient triage and treatment? *AJR* 2000; 175:99–103.

Dani R, Nogueira CED. Chronische kalzifzierende pankreatitis in Brasilien Eine analyse von 92 fallen. *Leber Magen Darm*. 1976; 6: 272-5.

Whitcomb DC. Mechanisms of Disease: advances in understanding the mechanisms leading to chronic pancreatitis. *Nature Clinical Practice Gastroenterology Hepatology*. 2004; 1:46-52.

Whitcomb DC. Genetic Aspects of Pancreatitis. *Annual Review of Medicine*. 2010; 61:213-24.

Deussing J. Cathepsin B and D are dispensable for major histocompatibility complex class II-mediated antigen presentation. *Proc Natl Academy Science USA*.1998; 95:4516–4521.

Diaconu BL, Ciobanu L, Mocan T, Pfützer RH, Scafaru MP, Acalovschi M, Singer MV, Schneider A. Investigation of the SPINK1 N34S mutation in Romanian patients with alcoholic chronic pancreatitis. A clinical analysis based on the criteria of the MANNHEIM classification. *Journal of Gastrointestinal Liver Dis*. 2009; 18:143-150.

Di Magno EP, Buxton JL, Regan PT, Hattery RR, Wilson DA, Suarez JR, Green PS. Ultrasonic endoscope. *Lancet*.1980; 1:629-31.

Di Magnoa MJ, Di Magno EP. Chronic pancreatitis *Current Opinion in Gastroenterology*. 2010; 26:490–498.

Donghui L, Maha A, Yanan, L. 5, 10-Methylenetetrahydrofolate Reductase Polymorphisms and the Risk of Pancreatic Cancer. *Cancer Epidemiology Biomarkers Prev*. 2005; 14:1470-1476.

Drenth JP, te MR, Jansen JB. Mutations in serine protease inhibitor Kazal type 1 are strongly associated with chronic pancreatitis. *Gut*. 2002; 50:687–92.

Duggan S, Sullivan OM, Feehan S, Ridgway P, Conlon K. Nutrition treatment of deficiency and malnutrition in chronic pancreatitis: a review. *Nutrition Clinical Practice*. 2010; 25:362-370.

Etemad B, Whitcomb DC. Chronic pancreatitis: diagnosis, classification, and new genetic developments. *Gastroenterology*. 2001; 120:682-707.

Expert Committee on the Diagnosis of Classification of Diabetes Mellitus. Report of the expert committee on the diagnosis of classification of diabetes mellitus. *Diabetes Care* 1997; 20: 1183-97.

Fanen P, Hasnain A. Cystic Fibrosis and CFTR Gene. Atlas Genetics Cytogenetics OncologyHaematol;2001. Availablefromhttp://Atlas GeneticsOncology.org/Educ/CistFibID300 2ES.Html, accessed on January 3, 2011.

Ferrone M, Raimondo M, Scolapio JS. Pancreatic enzyme pharmacotherapy. *Pharmacotherapy*. 2007; 27:910–920.

Figarella C, Miszczuk-Jamska B, Barrett A. Possible lysosomal activation of pancreatic zymogens. Activation of both human trypsinogens by cathepsin B and spontaneous acid. Activation of human trypsinogen-1. *Biology Chem Hoppe Seyler*.1988; 369:293–298.

Finkelberg DL, Sahani D, Deshpande V, Brugge WR. Autoimmune pancreatitis. *N England Journal of Medicine* 2006; 355:2670-6.

Fodinger, M., Molecular biology of 5, 10-methylenetetrahydrofolate reductase. *Nephrology*. 2000; 13:20-33.

Forsmark CE. Chronic pancreatitis. In: Feldman M, Freidman L, Sleisenger M, eds. *Gastrointestinal and Liver Disease*. Philadelphia: WB Saunders, 2002:953.

Chandak GR, Idris MM, Reddy DN, Bhaskar SS, Sriram PVJ, Singh L. Mutations in the pancreatic secretary trypsin inhibitor gene (PSTI/SPINK1) rather than the cationic trypsinogen gene (PRSS1) are significantly associated with tropical calcific pancreatitis. *Journal of Medical Genetics* 2002; 39:347–351.

Gadsby DC, Vergani P, Csanády L. The ABC protein turned chloride channel whose failure causes cystic fibrosis. *Nature*. 2006; 440: 477-83.

Garg PK, Khajuria R, Kabra M, Shastri SS. Association of SPINK1 gene mutation and CFTR gene polymorphisms in patients with pancreas divisum presenting with idiopathic pancreatitis. *Journal of Clinical Gastroenterology*.2009; 43:848-52.

Gąsiorowska A, Talar-Wojnarowska R, Czupryniak L. The prevalence of cationic trypsinogen (PRSS1) and serine protease inhibitor, Kazal type 1 (SPINK1) gene mutations in Polish patients with alcoholic and idiopathic chronic pancreatitis. *Digestive Disease Science*. 2011; 56: 894-901.

Geevarghese PJ. *Calcific Pancreatitis*. Bombay: Varghese Publishing House, 1985.

Geevarghese PJ. *Pancreatic diabetes*. Bombay: Popular Prakashan, 1968:110–115.

Geeverghese PJ, Kumarapilla V, Joseph MP, Pitchumoni CS. The diagnosis of pancreatogenous diabetes mellitus (A clinico-pathological study of one hundred cases of pancreatic calculi associated with diabetes mellitus). *Journal of Association Physicians India.* 1962; 10: 173-80.

Goodall JW, Pilbeam SJ. Diabetes in Nyasaland (Malawi). *Trans R Soc Tropical Medicine Hyg.* 1964; 58:575-8.

Gorelick F, Matovcik L. Lysosomal enzymes and pancreatitis. *Gastroenterology.* 1995; 109:620-5.

Goulden MR. The pain of chronic pancreatitis: a persistent clinical challenge. *British Journal of Pain* February 20, 2013:10.117.

Govindarajan M, Mohan V, Deepa R. Histopathology and immunohistochemistry of pancreatic islets in fibrocalculous pancreatic diabetes. *Diabetes Res Clin Pract.* 2001; 51:29.

Grant JP. Nutritional support in acute and chronic pancreatitis. *Surg Clinical North Am.* 2011; 91:805-20.

Haber PS, Norris MD, Apte MV, Rodgers SC, Norton ID, Pirola RC. Alcoholic pancreatitis and polymorphisms of the variable length polythymidine tract in the cystic fibrosis gene. *Alcohol Clinical Experimental Research.* 1999; 23:509–12.

Hai-Xia, C. Genetic Polymorphisms of Methylenetetrahydrofolate Reductase and Susceptibility to Colorectal Cancer. Asian Pacific. *J. Cancer Prev.* 2008; 9: 203-208.

Halangk W, Lerch MM, Brandt Nedelev B, Roth W, Ruthenbuerger M, Reinheckel T, et al. Role of cathepsin B in intracellular trypsinogen activation and the onset of acute pancreatitis. *Journal of Clinical Investigation.*2000; 106:773–81.

Hassan Z, Mohan V, Ali L, Allotey R, Barakat K, Faruque MO. SPINK1 is a susceptibility gene for fibrocalculous pancreatic diabetes in subjects from the Indian subcontinent. *American Journal of Human Genetics.* 2002; 71:964–8.

Hobbs, C.A. Polymorphisms in Genes Involved in Folate Metabolism as Maternal Risk Factors for Down syndrome. *Am. J. Human Genetics.* 2000, 67:623-630.

Horii A, Kobayashi T, Tomita N, Yamamoto T, Fukushige S, Murotsu T, Ogawa M, Mori T, Matsubara K. Primary structure of human pancreatic secretary trypsin inhibitor (PSTI) gene. *Biochemical Biophysical Research Community.* 1987; 149:635-41.

Howes N, Lerch MM, Green half W, Stocken DD, Ellis I, Simon P, Truninger K, Amman R, Cavallini G, Charnley RM, Uomo G, Delhaye M, Spicak J, Drumm B, Jansen J, Mountford R, Whitcomb DC, Neoptolemos JP. European Registry of Hereditary Pancreatitis and Pancreatic Cancer

(EUROPAC). Clinical and genetic characteristics of hereditary pancreatitis in Europe. *Clinical Gastroenterology Hepatology.* 2004; 2:252-61.

Huges D, Thilo Dork T, Stuhrmann M, Graham C. Mutation and haplotype analysis of the CFTR gene in atypically mild cystic fibrosis patients from Northern Ireland. *Journal of Medical Genetics* 2001; 38:136-139.

International Workshop on Types of Diabetes Peculiar to the Tropics. Consensus statement from the International Workshop on Types of Diabetes Peculiar to the Tropics, 17-19, October 1995, Cuttack, India. *Acta Diabetology Latina* 1996; 33: 62-64.

Ivan, N, Jelena D. MTHFR C677T polymorphism in chronic pancreatitis and pancreatic adenocarcinoma. *Cell. Biochemical. Function.*2008; 26: 659-663.

Kabra SK, Kabra M, Lodha R, Shastri S, Ghosh M, Pandey RM. Clinical profile and frequency of delta f508 mutation in Indian children with cystic fibrosis. *Indian Pediatric* 2003; 40: 612-9.

Kahl S, Glasbrenner B, Leodolter A, Pross M, Schulz HU, Malfertheiner P. EUS in the diagnosis of early chronic pancreatitis: a prospective follow-up study. *Gastrointestinal Endoscopy.*2002; 55:507-11.

Kaneko K, Nagasaki Y, Furukawa T, Mizutamari H, Sato A, Masamune A. Analysis of the human pancreatic secretary trypsin inhibitor (PSTI) gene mutations in Japanese patients with chronic pancreatitis. *Journal of Hum Genet.*2001; 46:293–7.

Kaneto H, Katakami N, Kawamori D, Miyatsuka T, Sakamoto K, Matsuoka TA, Matsuhisa M, and Yamasaki Y. Involvement of oxidative stress in the pathogenesis of diabetes. *Antioxidant Redox Signal.* 2007; 9: 355–66.

Kazal LA, Sopicer DS, Brahinski RA. Isolation of a crystalline trypsin inhibitor-anticoagulant protein from pancreas. *Journal of the American Chemistry Society.*1948; 70:3034-3040.

Keim V, Teich N, Moessner J. Clinical value of a new fecal elastase test for detection of chronic pancreatitis. *Clinical Lab.* 2003; 49:209-15.

Kiesewetter S, Macek S Jr, Davis C. A mutation in CFTR produces different phenotypes depending on chromosomal background. *Nat Genetics.*1993; 5:274-280.

Kini MG. Multiple pancreatic calculi with chronic pancreatitis. *Br Journal of Surgery.* 1937; 25:705.

Kinnear TWG. The pattern of diabetes mellitus in a Nigerian teaching hospital. *East African Med J* 1963; 40:288-94.

Kiraly O, Boulling A, Witt H, Marechal Le, Chen JM, Rosendahl J, Battaggia C, Wartmann T, Sahin-Toth M, Ferec C. Signal peptide variants that impair secretion of pancreatic secretary trypsin inhibitor (SPINK1) cause autosomal dominant hereditary pancreatitis. *Human Mutation.* 2007; 28:469-76.

Klöppel G, Maillet B. Chronic pancreatitis: evolution of the disease. *Hepatology Gastroenterology.*1991; 38: 408-412.

Kume K, Masamune A, Mizutamari H, Kaneko K, Kikuta K, Satoh M, et al. Mutations in the serine protease inhibitor Kazal Type 1 (SPINK1) gene in Japanese patients with pancreatitis. *Pancreatology.*2005; 5:354–60.

Kume K, Masamune A, Kikuta K, Shimosegawa T. [-215G>A; IVS3+2T>C] mutation in the SPINK1 gene causes exon 3 skipping and loss of the trypsin binding site. *Gut.*2006; 55:1214.

Kuno A, Yamada T, Masuda K, Ogawa K, Sogawa M, Nakamura S. Angiotensin-converting enzyme inhibitor attenuates pancreatic inflammation and fibrosis in male Wistar Bonn/Kobori rats *Gastroenterology.*2003; 124:1010–9.

Kuwata K, Hirota M, Sugita H, Kai M, Hayashi N, Nakamura M, Matsuura T, Adachi N, Nishimori I, Ogawa M. Genetic mutations in exons 3 and 4 of the pancreatic secretary trypsin inhibitor in patients with pancreatitis. *Journal of Gastroenterology.*2001; 36:612-618.

Kuwata K, Hirota M, Shimizu H, Nakae M, Nishihara S, Takimoto A. Functional analysis of recombinant pancreatic secretary trypsin inhibitor protein with amino-acid substitution. *Journal of Gastroenterology.*2002; 37:928–34.

Lankisch PG, Seidensticker F, Lohr-Happe A. The course of pain is the same in alcohol and non-alcohol- induced chronic pancreatitis. *Pancreas.* 1995; 10:338.

Layer P, Keller J. Lipase supplementation therapy: standards, alternatives, and perspectives. *Pancreas.*2003;26:1–7.

Bodic Le, Bignon JD, Raguenes O, Mercier B, Georgelin T, Schnee M, Soulard F, Gagne K, Bonneville F, Muller JY, Bachner L, Ferec C. The hereditary pancreatitis gene maps to long arm of chromosome 7. *Hum Mol Genet.* 1996; 5:549-54.

Lebo RV, Grody WW. Variable penetrance and expressivity of the splice 5T sequences in the cystic fibrosis gene. *Genetic Testing.* 2007; 11:32-44.

Lempinen M, Paju A, Kemppainen E, Smura T, Kylänpää ML, Nevanlinna H, Stenman J, Stenman UH. Mutations N34S and P55S of the SPINK1 gene in patients with chronic pancreatitis or pancreatic cancer and in healthy subjects: a report from Finland. *Scand J Gastroenterology.* 2005; 40:225-230.

Lee JH, Choi JH, Namkung W, Hanrahan JW, Chang J, Song SY, Park SW, Kim DS, Yoon JH, Suh Y, Jang IJ, Nam JH, Kim SJ, Cho MO, Lee JE, Kim KH, Lee MG. A haplotype-based molecular analysis of CFTR mutations associated with respiratory and pancreatic diseases. *Hum Mol Genet* 2003; 12: 2321-32.

Leung PS, Chappell MC. A local pancreatic renin-angiotensin system: endocrine and exocrine roles. *International Journal of Biochemical. Cell Biol.*2003; 35:834–46.

Lin Y, Tamakoshi A, Matsunao S. Nationwide epidemiological survey of chronic pancreatitis in Japan. *Journal of Gastroenterology.* 2000; 35:136-41.

Lowenfels AB, Maisonneuve P, DiMagno EP, Elitsur Y, Gates LK Jr, Perrault J, Whitcomb DC. Hereditary pancreatitis and the risk of pancreatic cancer. International Hereditary Pancreatitis Study Group. *Journal of Natl Cancer Inst.* 1997; 89:442-6.

Lowenfels AB, Maisonneuve P, Whitcomb DC, Lerch MM, Dimagno EP. Cigarette smoking as a risk factor for pancreatic cancer in patients with hereditary pancreatitis. *JAMA.* 2001; 286:169–70.

Lowenfels AB, Maisonneuve P. Risk factors for pancreatic cancer. *Journal of Cellular Biochemical.*2005; 95:649-56.

Mahurkar S, Idris MM, Reddy DN, Bhaskar S, Rao GV, Thomas V. Association of cathepsin B gene polymorphisms with tropical calcific pancreatitis. *Gut.* 2006;55:1270–5.

Maire F, Bienvenu T, Ngukam A, Hammel P, Ruszniewski P, Lévy P. Frequency of CFTR gene mutations in idiopathic pancreatitis. *Gastroenterology of Clinical Biology.* 2003; 27:398-402.

Malats N, Casals T, Porta M, Guarner L, Estivill X, Real FX. Cystic fibrosis transmembrane regulator (CFTR) DeltaF508 mutation and 5T allele in patients with chronic pancreatitis and exocrine pancreatic cancer. PANKRAS II Study Group. *Gut.2001*; 48:70–4.

March bank, T, Freeman T.C, Play ford R.J. Human pancreatic secretary trypsin inhibitor. *Digestion.* 1998; 59:167–174.

Marks IN, Bank S, Berk JE, Haubrich WS, Kalser MH, Roth JLA, Schaffner F, Bockus eds. Aetiology, clinical aspects, and medical management. *Gastroenterology* 1985:4020-40.

Matsubayashi H, Fukushima N, Sato N, Brune K, Canto M, Yeo CJ, Hruban RH, Kern SE, Goggins M. Polymorphisms of SPINK1 N34S and CFTR in patients with sporadic and familial pancreatic cancer. *Cancer Biology and Therapy*. 2003;2:652-655.

McMillan DE, Geevarghese PJ. Dietary cyanide and tropical malnutrition diabetes. *Diabetes Care.*1979; 2:202–8.

Mergener K, Baillie J. Chronic pancreatitis. *Lancet.*1997; 350:1379-85.

Miao X, Xing D, Tan W. Susceptibility to gastric cardia adenocarcinoma and genetic polymorphisms in methylenetetrahydrofolate reductase in an at-risk Chinese population. *Cancer Epidemiology Biomarkers Prev.* 2002;11:1454–1458.

Michael J, Coffey L, Chee Y. Pancreatitis in Cystic Fibrosis and CFTR-Related Disorder. In: *Acute pancreatitis.* 2012; 67-90.

Midha S, Khajuria R, Shastri S, Kabra M, Garg PK. Idiopathic chronic pancreatitis in India: phenotypic characterisation and strong genetic susceptibility due to SPINK1 and CFTR gene mutations. *Gut.*2010; 59:800-7.

Mittal N, Mehrotra R, Agarwal G, Rajeshwari J, Choudhuri G, Sikora S. The clinical spectrum of fibrocalculous pancreatic diabetes in North India. *Natl Medical J India.*2002; 15:327–31.

Mohan V, Chari ST, Hitman GA, Suresh S, Madanagopalan N, Ramachandran A. Familial aggregation in tropical fibrocalculous pancreatic diabetes. *Pancreas.*1989; 4:690–3.

Mohan V, Premlatha G. Fibrocalculus pancreatic diabetes. *International Journal of Diabetes.*1995; 3:71-82.

Mohan V, Farooq S, Deepa M. Prevalence of fibrocalculous pancreatic diabetes in Chennai in South India. *JOP*. 2008; 9:489-492.

Mohan V, Premalatha G. Fibrocalculous pancreatic diabetes. *International Journal of Diabetes.* 1995;3:71-82.

Monaghan KG, Jackson CE, Ku Kuruga DL, Feldman GL. Mutation analysis of the cystic fibrosis and cationic trypsinogen genes in patients with alcohol-related pancreatitis. *American Journal of Medical Genetics.*2000; 9:120–4.

Monique H.M, Derikx, Joost P.H. Drenth. Genetic factors in chronic pancreatitis; implications for diagnosis, management and prognosis. *Best Practice & Research Clinical Gastroenterology.*2010; 251–270.

Ahmed N, Corey M, Forstner G, Zielenski J, Tsui L, Tullis Ellis E, Durie P. Molecular consequences of cystic fibrosis transmembrane regulator (CFTR) gene mutations in the exocrine pancreas. *Gut* 2003; 52:1159–1164.

Malats N, Casals T, Porta M, Guarner L, Estivill X, Real FX. PANKRAS II Study Group. Cystic fibrosis transmembrane regulator (CFTR) ΔF508 mutation and 5T allele in patients with chronic pancreatitis and exocrine pancreatic cancer. *Gut* 2001; 48:70-74.

Nagalotimath SJ. Pancreatic pathology in pancreatic calcification with diabetes. In: Podolsky S, Viswanathan M, eds. *Secondary diabetes: the spectrum of diabetic syndromes.* New York: Raven Press, 1980:117–45.

Nagalotimath SJ. Pancreatic in Karnataka. A note on pathology. In: Balakrishnan V, ed. chronic pancreatitis in India. *Trivandrum: Indian Society of Pancreatology.* 1986:105-110.

Nagarathnam N, Gunawardane KRW. *Etiological factors in pancreatic calcification in Ceylon. Digestion.*1972; 5: 9-16.5.

Nair B. Pathology of tropical calcific pancreatitis. In: Kumar N, Acharya SK, eds. *Tropical calcific pancreatitis.* Kerala: Roussel Scientific Institute. 1994:83–90.

Oruc Nevin, Papachristou Georgios I, Avula Haritha, Slivka Adam, Lamb Janette, Whitcomb David C. Angiotensin-converting enzyme gene DD genotype neither increases susceptibility to acute pancreatitis nor influences disease severity. *International Hepatology Pancreato-Biliary Association.*2009; 11:45-49.

Oruc Nevin, Papachristou Georgios I, Avula Haritha, Slivka Adam, Lamb Janette, Whitcomb David C. The Functional Angiotensin Converting Enzyme Gene I/D Polymorphism do not Alter Susceptibility to Chronic Pancreatitis. *JOP.* 2004; 5:457-463.

Niederau C, Grendell JH. Diagnosis of chronic pancreatitis. *Gastroenterology.*1985; 88:1973.

Nikolić A, Dinić J, Radojković D, Lukić S, Popović D, Ugljesić M, Knezević S. CFTR F508DEL mutation and 5T allele in patients with chronic pancreatitis and pancreatic adenocarcinoma. *Acta Chir Iugosl.* 2011; 58:43-7.

Noone PG, Zhou Z, Silverman LM, Jowell PS, Knowles MR, Cohn JA. Cystic fibrosis gene mutations and pancreatitis risk: relation to epithelial ion transport and trypsin inhibitor gene mutations. *Journal of Cystic Fibrosis.*2001; 121:1310-19.

Olurin EO, Olurin O. Pancreatic calcification: a report of 45 cases. *Br Med J* 1969; 4:5349.

Ooi C.Y, Dupuis A, Ellis L, Jarvi K, Martin S, Gonska T, Dorfman R, Kortan P, Solomon M, Tullis E, Durie P.R. Comparing the American and

European diagnostic guidelines for cystic fibrosis: same disease, different language? *Thorax* 2012; 67:7 618-624.

Ota Y, Masamune A, Inui K, Kume K, Shimosegawa T, Kikuyama M. Phenotypic variability of the homozygous IVS3+2T>C mutation in the serine protease inhibitor Kazal type 1(SPINK1) gene in patients with chronic pancreatitis. *Tohoku J Exp Med.* 2010; 221:197-201.

Pandol SJ. San Rafael (CA): Sciences. The Exocrine Pancreas. 2010.

Pandya A, Blanton SH, Landa B, Javaheri R, Melvin E, Nance WE, Markello T. Linkage studies in a large kindred with hereditary pancreatitis confirms mapping of the gene to a 16-cM region on 7q. *Genomics.*1996; 38:227-30.

Papapetrou C, Lynch S.A, Burn J, Edwards, Y.H. Methylenetetrahydrofolate reductase and neural tube defects. *Lancet.*1996; 15: 348-358.

Papita R. Secular trends of fibrocalculous pancreatic diabetes and diabetes secondary to alcoholic chronic pancreatitis at a tertiary care diabetes centre in South India. *Journal of Pancreas.* 2012; 13:205-209.

Parsa I, Marsh W, Fitzgerald P. Pancreas acinar cell differentiation, Effects of methyl donors and homocysteine. *Fed Proc.*1972; 31:166–175.

Pasricha PJ. Unraveling the mystery of pain in chronic pancreatitis. *Gastroenterology Hepatology.* 2012; 7:235-240

Peach MJ. Renin-angiotensin system: biochemistry and mechanisms of action. *Physiology Review.* 1977; 57:313-70.

Peadar G.N, Charles A.P, Zhou Z, Michael R.K. "Lung Disease Associated with the IVS8 5T Allele of the CFTR Gene". *American Journal of Respiratory and Critical Care Medicine.* 2000; 61:1919-1924.

Peláez-Luna M, Canizales S, Tusié-Luna M T, Robles-Díaz G. The Homozygous N34s Spink-1 Mutation Is Not Sufficient to Produce Acute or Chronic Pancreatitis. Report of a Mexican Family With Spink-1 N34s Mutation. *Pancreas.*2010; 31:462-467.

Perri F, Piepoli A, Stanziale P, Merla A, Zelante L, Andriulli A. Mutation analysis of the cystic fibrosis transmembrane conductance regulator (CFTR) gene, the cationic trypsinogen (PRSS1) gene, and the serine protease inhibitor, Kazal type 1 (SPINK1) gene in patients with alcoholic chronic pancreatitis. *European Journal of Human Genetics.* 2003; 11:687-92.

Pezzilli R, Morselli Labate AM, Fantini L, Gullo L, Corinaldesi R. Quality of life and clinical indicators for chronic pancreatitis patients in a 2-year follow-up study. *Pancreas.*2007; 34:191-6.

Pezzilli R. Chronic pancreatitis: maldigestion, intestinal ecology and intestinal inflammation. *World J Gastroenterology.*2009; 15(14):1673–1676.

Pitchumoni CS, Viswanathan KV, Geevarghese PJ, Banks PA. Ultrastructure and elemental composition of human pancreatic calculi. *Pancreas* 1987; 2:152–8.

Pitchumoni CS, Jain NK, Lowenfels AB, et al. Chronic cyanide poisoning:unifying concept for alcoholic and tropical pancreatitis. *Pancreas.* 1988; 3:220-2.

Pitchumoni CS. Special problems of tropical pancreatitis. *Clinical Gastroenterology.*1984; 13:941-59.

Pitchumoni CS. Familial pancreatitis. In: Pai KN, Soman CR, Varghese R, Eds. Pancreatic Diabetes. *Trivandrum: Geo Printers.* 1970: 46-8.

Prasad R, Sharma H, Kaur G. Molecular Basis of Cystic Fibrosis Disease: An Indian Perspective. *Ind J Clin Biochem* 2010; 25: 335–41.

Raffaele Pezzilli. Pain in Chronic Pancreatitis: From the Bench to the Bedside. *Journal of Pancreas.*2012; 13:245-246.

Ravnik-Glavac M, Dean M, Sant'Agnese P, Chernick M, Kozelj M, Krizman I, Glavac D. Evidence that hereditary pancreatitis is genetically heterogeneous disorder. *Pflugers. Arch.* 2000; 439-443.

Reboul MP, Laharie D, Amouretti M, Lacombe D, Iron A. Isolated idiopathic chronic pancreatitis associated with a compound heterozygosity for two mutations of the CFTR gene. *Gastroenterology Clinical Biology.* 2003; 27:821-824.

Reddy DN, Prasad SS. Genetic basis of chronic pancreatitis in Asia Pacific region. *Journal of Gastroenterology and Hepatology.* 2011; 2:2-5.

Rigat B, Hubert C, Alhenc-Gelas F, Cambien F, Corvol P, Soubier F. An insertion/deletion polymorphism in the angiotensin I-converting enzyme gene accounting for half of variance of serum enzyme levels. *Journal of Clinical Invest.*1990; 86:1343–6.

Riordan J. R, Rommens J. M, Kerem B, Alon N, Rozmahel R., Grzelczak Z, Zielenski J, Lok S, Plavsic N, Chou J. L, Drumm M. L, Iannuzzi M. C, Collins F. S, Tsui L.-C. "Identification of the cystic fibrosis gene: cloning and characterization of complementary DNA." *Science.*1989; 245: 1066-1073.

Mitchell RMS, Byrne MF, Baillie J. Pancreatitis. *The Lancet.* 2003; 9367:1447-145.

Rossi L, Whitcomb DC, Ehrlich GD, Gorry MC, Parvin S, Sattar S, Ali L, Azad Khan AK, Gyr N. Lack of R117H mutation in the cationic trypsinogen gene in patients with tropical calcific pancreatitis from Bangladesh. *Pancreas.*1998; 17:278-80.

Ryter SW, Kim HP, Hoetzel A, Park JW, Nakahira K, Wang X, and Choi AM. Mechanisms of cell death in oxidative stress. *Antioxidant Redox Signal* 9: 49–89, 2007.

Saluja A, Hashimoto S, Saluja M, Powers RE, Meldolesi J, Steer ML. Subcellular redistribution of lysosomal enzymes during caerulein-induced pancreatitis. *Am J Physiol* 1987; 253:G508-16.

Schneider A, Suman A, Rossi L, Barmada MM, Beglinger C, Parvin S. SPINK1/PSTI mutations are associated with tropical pancreatitis and type II diabetes mellitus in Bangladesh. *Gastroenterology.*2002; 123:1026–30.

Schneider A, Suman A, Rossi L, Barmada MM, Beglinger C, Parvin S. SPINK1/PSTI mutations are associated with tropical pancreatitis and type II diabetes mellitus in Bangladesh. *Gastroenterology.*2002; 123:1026–30.

Schneider, J.A. and Rees, D.C., Worldwide distribution of a common methylenetetrahydrofolate reductase mutation. *American Journal of Human Genetics.*1998, 62:1258–1260.

Schultz AC, Moore PB, Geevarghese PJ. X-ray diffraction studies of pancreatic calculi associated with nutritional pancreatitis. *Digestive Disease Science.*1986; 31:476–80.

Seno T, Harada H, Ochi K, Tanaka J, Matsumoto S, Choudhury R, et al. Serum levels of six pancreatic enzymes as related to the degree of renal dysfunction. *American Journal of Gastroenterology* 1995; 90:2002-5.

Midha Shallu, Khajuria Rajni, Garg Kumar Pramod, Kabra Madhulika. Idiopathic chronic pancreatitis in India: phenotypic characterisation and strong genetic susceptibility due to SPINK1 and CFTR gene mutations. *Gut* 2010; 59:800-807.

Sharer N, Schwartz M, Malone G. Mutations of the cystic fibrosis gene in patients with chronic pancreatitis. *New England Journal of Medicine.*1998; 339:645-652.

Sharma N, Singh M, Kaur G, Thapa BR, Prasad R. Identification and characterization of CFTR gene mutation in Indian CF patients. *Annals of Human Genetics.* 2009;76: 26–33.

Shastri SS, Kabra M, Kabra SK, Pandey RM, Menon PS. Characterisation of mutations and genotype-phenotype correlation in cystic fibrosis: *Experience from Indian Journal of Cystic Fibrosis* 2008; 7: 110-5.

Shimosegawa T, Kume K, Masamune A. SPINK1 gene mutations and pancreatitis in Japan. *Journal of Gastroenterology and Hepatology.* 2006; 47-51.

Singh S, Choudhuri G, Kumar R, Agarwal S. Association of 5,10 methylenetetrahydrofolate Reductase C667T polymorphism in susceptibility to tropical chronic pancreatitis in north Indian population. *Cellular Molecular Biol.* 2012; 5 8:122-127.

Singh Shweta, Choudhuri Gourdas and Agarwal Sarita. Genetic and Environmental Attributes of Chronic Pancreatitis. *British Journal of Applied Science and Technology.* 2013;3:206-213.

Singh S, Kumar R, Choudhuri G, Agarwal S. Chronic Pancreatitis: A new pathophysiology. *Indian Journal of Human Genetics.*2012;18:380- 382.

Snabboon T, Plengpanich W, Sridama V, Sunthornyothin S, Suwanwalaikorn S, Khovidhunkit W.A SPINK1 gene mutation in a Thai patient with fibrocalculous pancreatic diabetes. *Southeast Asian J Tropical Medical Public Health* 2006; 37:559–62.

Somogyi L, Ross SO, Cintron M, Toskes PP. Comparison of biologic porcine secretin, synthetic porcine secretin, and synthetic human secretin in pancreatic function testing. *Pancreas* 2003; 27:230-4.

Song C, Xing D, Tan W. Methylenetetrahydrofolate reductase polymorphisms increase risk of esophageal squamous cell carcinoma in a Chinese population. *Cancer Research.*2001; 61:3272–3275.

Sonnet H, Brisbois P, Bastin JP. Chronic pancreatitis with calcifications in Congolese Bantus. *Tropical Geogr Med* 1966; 18:97-113.

Spielman R.S, McGinnis R.E, Ewens W.J. Transmission test for linkage disequilibrium: the insulin gene region and insulin-dependent diabetes mellitus (IDDM). *Am J. Hum. Genet.*52, 506–516 (1993).

Steer ML, Waxman I, Freedman S. Chronic pancreatitis. *N Engl J Med* 1995; 332:1482.

Stevenson, R.E., Schwartz, C.E., Du, Y-Z., and Adams, M.J., Differences in methylenetetrahydrofolate reductase genotype frequencies between whites and blacks. *American Journal of Human Genetics.*1999; 60:229–23.

Strom CM. Cystic fibrosis screening using the college panel: platform comparison and lessons learned from the first 20,000 samples. Genetics Medicine.2002; 4:289–96.

Stroth U, Unger T. The renin angiotensin system and its receptors. *J Cardiovascular Pharmacol* 1999; 33:S21-8.

Suzuki T, Matsuo K, Sawaki A, Mizuno N, Hiraki A, Kawase T, Watanabe M, Nakamura T, Yamao K, Tajima K, Tanaka H. Alcohol Drinking and One-Carbon Metabolism-Related Gene Polymorphisms on Pancreatic Cancer Risk. *Cancer Epidemiology Biomarkers Prev.* 2008, 17:2742-2747.

Talamini G, Bassi C. Alcohol and smoking as risk factors in chronic pancreatitis and pancreatic cancer. *Digestive Disease Science.* 1999; 44:1303-1311.

Teich N, Rosendahl J, Toth M, Mossner J, Sahin-Toth M. Mutations of human cationictrypsinogen (PRSS1) and chronic pancreatitis. *Human Mutation.*2006; 27:721-30.

Thomas PG, Augustine P, Ramesh H, Rangabashyam N. Observation and surgical management of tropical pancreatitis in Kerala and southern India. *World J Surgery.*1990; 14:32-42.

Thread gold J, Green half W, Ellis I, Howes N, Lerch MM, Simon P. The N34S mutation of SPINK1 (PSTI) is associated with a familial pattern of idiopathic chronic pancreatitis but does not cause the disease. *Gut* 2002; 50: 675–81.

Truninger K, Witt H, Kock J, Kage A, Seifert B, Ammann RW, Blum HE, Becker M. Mutations of the serine protease inhibitor, Kazal type 1 in patients with idiopathic chronic pancreatitis. *American Journal of Gastroenterology.* 2002; 97: 1133–1137.

Truninger K, Kock J, Wirth HP, Muellhaupt B, Arnold C, von WF. Trypsinogen gene mutations in patients with chronic or recurrent acute pancreatitis. *Pancreas.* 2001; 22:18–23.

Tsui, Lap-Chee."CFTR Mutation Table." http://www.genet.sickkids.on.ca/cftr. Cystic fibrosis mutation database. Cystic Fibrosis Genetic Analysis Consortium 2001.

Tzetis M, Kaliakatsos M, Fotoulaki M, Papatheodorou A, Doudounakis S. Contribution of the CFTR gene, the pancreatic secretary trypsin inhibitor gene (SPINK1) and the cationic trypsinogen gene (PRSS1) to the etiology of recurrent pancreatitis. *Clinical genetics.*2007; 71:451:457.

UlvikA, Evensen E.T, Lien E.A. Smoking, folate and methylenetetrahydro folatereductase status as interactive determinants of adenomatous and hyperplastic polyps of colorectum. *American Journal of Medical Genetics.*2001; 101:246–254.

Vander P.N.M.J., Eskes, T.K.A.B., Blom, H.J. Is the common 677CT mutation in the methylenetetrahydrofolate reductase gene a risk factor for neural tube defects? *A meta analysis. Q. J. Med.* 1997; 90:111–115.

Balakrishnan V, Nair Prem, Radhakrishnan Laxmi, Narayanan VA. *Tropical pancreatitis a distinct entity or merely a type of chronic pancreatitis.* Indian Society of Gastroenterology. 2006.

Watanabe O, Baccino FM, Steer ML, Meldolesi J. Supramaximal caerulein stimulation and ultrastructure of rat pancreatic acinar cell: early morphological changes during development of experimental pancreatitis. *American Journal of Physiology.* 1984; 246:457–67.

Weiss FU, Simon P, Witt H, Mayerle J, Hlouschek V. SPINK1 mutation and phenotypic expression in patients with pancreatitis associated with trypsinogen mutation. *Journal of Medical Genetics.*2003; 40:43.

Whitcomb DC, Gorry MC, Preston RA, Furey W, Sossenheimer MJ, Ulrich CD, Martin SP, Gates LK Jr, Amann ST, Toskes PP, Liddle R, McGrath K, Uomo G, Post JC, Ehrlich GD. Hereditary pancreatitis is caused by a mutation in the cationic trypsinogen gene. *Nature Genetics.* 1996;14: 141-5.

Whitcomb DC, Preston RA, Aston CE, Sossenheimer MJ, Barua PS, Zhang Y, Wong-Chong A, White GJ, Wood PG, Gates LK Jr, Ulrich C, Martin SP, Post JC, Ehrlich GD. A gene for hereditary pancreatitis maps to chromosome 7q35. *Gastroenterology.* 1996a; 110:1975-80.

Whitcomb DC, Gorry MC, Preston RA, Furey W, Sossenheimer MJ, Ulrich CD, Martin SP, Gates LK Jr, Amann ST, Toskes PP, Liddle R, McGrath K, Uomo G, Post JC, Ehrlich GD. Hereditary pancreatitis is caused by a mutation in the cationic trypsinogen gene. *Nature Genetics.* 1996b; 14:141-5.

Wiersema MJ, Hawes RH, Lehman GA, Kochman ML, Sherman S, Kopecky KK. Prospective evaluation of endoscopic ultrasonography and endoscopic retrograde cholangiopancreatography in patients with chronic abdominal pain of suspected pancreatic origin. *Endoscopy.*1993; 25:555-64.

Witt H, Luck W, Becker M. A signal peptide cleavage site mutation in the cationic trypsinogen gene is strongly associated with chronic pancreatitis. *Gastroenterology.* 1999; 117:7-10.

Witt H, Luck W, Hennies HC, Claßen M, Kage A, Laß U. Mutations in the gene encoding mutations in the gene encoding the serine protease inhibitor, Kazal type 1 are associated with chronic pancreatitis. *Nature Genetics.*2000; 25:213–6.

Witt H, Apte MV, Keim V, Wilson JS. Chronic pancreatitis: challenges and advances in pathogenesis, genetics, diagnosis, and therapy. *Gastroenterology.*2007; 132:155773.

Witt H, LuckW, Becker M, Bohmig M, Kage A, Truninger K. Mutation in the SPINK1 trypsin inhibitor gene, alcohol use, and chronic pancreatitis. *JAMA.* 2001;285:2716–7.

Witt H, Luck W, Hennies HC, Classen M, Kage A, Lass U, Landt O, Becker M. Mutations in the gene encoding the serine protease inhibitor, Kazal type 1 are associated with chronic pancreatitis. *Nature Genetics.* 2000; 25: 213-216.

WHO study group report on diabetes mellitus? *WHO Technical Report series* No.727. Geneva. 1985.

Zuidema PJ. Calcification and cirrhosis of the pancreas in patients with deficient nutrition. *Doc Med Geography Trop Amsterdam.* 1955; 5:229.

Zuidema PJ. Cirrhosis and disseminated calcification of the pancreas in patients with malnutrition. *Tropical Geogr Med.* 1959; 11:70-4.

Shweta Singh, Ravindra Kumar, Gourdas Choudhuri, Sarita Agarwal. Chronic Pancreatitis: A new Pathophysiology. *Indian Journal of Human Genetics.*2012; 18:380- 382.

Shally Awasthi, Nutan Maurya, Sarita Agarwal, Pratibha Dixit, Muthuswamy Srinivasan, Shweta Singh. Association of CFTR gene mutation with bronchial asthma and its severity in Indian children: A case-control study. *Annals of Human Biology.* 2012; 39(2):113-21.

Shweta Singh, Ravindra Kumar Gourdas Choudhuri, Sarita Agarwal. Association of 5, 10 Methylenetetrahydrofolate Reductase C677T polymorphism in susceptibility to Tropical Chronic Pancreatitis. *Cellular and Molecular Biology.* 2012;58(1): 122-127.

Shweta Singh, Gourdas Choudhuri, Sarita Agarwal. Genetic and Environmental Attributes of Chronic Pancreatitis. *British Journal of Applied Science and Technology.* 2013; 3(2):206-213.

Shweta Singh, Ashok Kumar, Sarita Agarwal. Genetic insight of Schizophrenia: Past and Future perspectives. *Gene.* 2013 Oct 17. : S0378-1119(13)01344-9.

Srinivasan Muthuswamy, Sarita Agarwal, Shweta Singh, Pratibha Dixit, Nutan Maurya, Shally Awasthi, Gourdas Choudhuri. Spectrum and Distribution of CFTR gene mutation in Asthma and Chronic Pancreatitis cases in North Indian Population *Gene.* 2014 (Ahead of publication).

Shweta Singh, Gourdas Choudhuri, Sarita Agarwal. Frequency of CFTR, SPINK1and CATHEPSINB gene mutation in north Indian Population: connections between genetics and clinical data. *The Scientific World Journal.*2014 (Ahead of publication)

INDEX

A

B

C

D

E

F

G

H

I

N

O

P